BIRTH&SEX

SHEILA KITZINGER

BIRTH & SEX

The power and the passion

pinter
&
martin

Birth & Sex: The Power and the Passion

First published by Pinter & Martin Ltd 2012

ISBN 978-1-78066-050-9

British Library Cataloguing-in-Publication Data
A catalogue record for this book is available from the British Library.

Set in Minion

Line illustrations on pages 105–110 by Jonathan Meakin
Editor Debbie Kennett
Index by Helen Bilton

Printed and bound in the UK by TJ International Ltd, Padstow, Cornwall

This book has been printed on paper that is sourced and harvested from sustainable forests and is FSC accredited.

Pinter & Martin Ltd
6 Effra Parade
London SW2 1PS

www.pinterandmartin.com

www.sheilakitzinger.com

Dedicated to Polly Kitzinger,
with thanksgiving for her strong
feminist commitment and vibrant living.

CONTENTS

INTRODUCTION:
WHY I WRITE ABOUT BIRTH AND SEX

I was in a state of postnatal euphoria in January 1961. My fourth child was newborn. Like the others, it had been a home birth – and she was in bed beside me in a room scented with hyacinths, in our cottage outside Oxford. I decided that I wanted to write about the joy of birth, and help other women discover it.

Polly was waking at around five in the morning for a breastfeed and then lay contentedly on the bed gazing around at her new world. So I started to write *The Experience of Childbirth*. Writing early in the morning, in the first light of dawn, has stayed a habit – a quiet, peaceful time when my mind is still rich with waking thoughts, ideas, phrases. That first draft only took me six weeks. Then I read it through aloud (that was important, I think, because I wanted to speak to women in my own voice, not to harangue them), and amended it over another few weeks.

The challenge I faced was to create a language to convey the multi-faceted sensations of labour and birth, physical and emotional, to find words for the rush of energy as contractions squeezed the uterus, and the power that built mountains was released in your body, for the feeling as the baby's head crowned as if in a ring of fire, and the birth passion.

I have been criticised for describing birth-giving in terms of sex, imposing on women a compulsory sexual performance – birth with orgasm. But for me personally it was an intense psychosexual experience. This is not surprising, since both childbirth and lactation involve the same hormones as in sexual arousal.

My colleagues in the National Childbirth Trust (NCT) were often sceptical about this. The lovely Betty Parsons, antenatal teacher to celebrities, also taught Prince Charles and Princess Diana. He was an enthusiastic advocate of her birth education, and is said to have invited her to teach relaxation to Her Majesty the Queen. He hosted her 80th birthday at St James's Palace. When told (erroneously) that her fellow birth guru Sheila Kitzinger had suggested that the moment of birth could be compared to an orgasm, Betty told her class: 'Well. Honeys, if that's an orgasm, then keep me out of bed'.[1]

Nothing like *The Experience of Childbirth* had been published before. Grantly Dick-Read had written *Childbirth Without Fear*.[2] That was from a kindly male doctor's point of view. I admired him very much. He introduced fresh insight on birth. But sexual passion was nothing to do with it. He did not describe the amazing energy that poured through a woman's body. And he believed he had said the last word on the subject. He and his wife Jess were staying with us and over breakfast I got talking about research that I considered important. He was taking the top off a boiled egg, put down his spoon, and said firmly, 'I have done all the research that is necessary'.

He taught that birth 'shouldn't hurt' if the mother relaxed. But of course it did! The pain was a side-effect of the creative process, muscles tightening and stretching as the baby's head pressed down to be born – positive pain, pain with a purpose. He had photographs, too, but the women's faces were all stamped with black rectangles so that they couldn't possibly be recognised.

In France psychoprophylaxis – claimed to be *'accouchement sans douleur'* – was the latest fashion. An American, Marjorie Karmel, wrote *Thank you, Dr Lamaze* – to my mind a sycophantic book extolling the benefits of his method of strict training of breathing and relaxation.[3] It was an enthusiastic instruction manual. If a woman obeyed his teachings she 'should' have no pain. If she did feel pain, however, it was evidence that she had not conformed to the 'correct' number of huffs and puffs, did not hold her breath long enough when pushing, failed to practise assiduously, and lacked commitment. I was fed up with women being blamed for everything that happened to them.

I had no agent, but knew that the firm of Victor Gollancz was innovative, radical and idealistic. I sent the manuscript off to Victor, with a few photographs taken by Uwe, my husband, of me giving birth, breathing my way through contractions, smiling as I reached down to stroke a glistening head that had just emerged, and cradling a naked baby against my breasts. My brother-in-law, Hilary Rubinstein, worked with Victor Gollancz then. Victor called him to his office and announced, apparently with shocked disbelief, 'I have photographs of your sister-in-law's private parts on my desk.'

I am grateful to them for their courage. They decided to go ahead and publish. It was clear sailing from then on. The editor suggested a few minor amendments. Otherwise, the book came out in 1962 exactly as I wrote it in that post-birth milky, glowing 'babymoon'.

There are hotels that now advertise 'babymoons' for mothers, fathers and babies. But when I intended to focus on feelings that follow spontaneously on an intense and ecstatic psychosexual experience of birth, it was not my idea that anyone should make money out of it.

The Observer serialised three chapters of *The Experience of Childbirth*, the first extract taking up the whole front page of the supplement. With four children under five, I had no spare time. Any career as a social anthropologist was certainly on hold. But now I was a writer! *The Experience of Childbirth* was later sold to Penguin and went through 23 impressions with them. It has been published in various languages, and sold well over a million copies. It is still in print in a revised form as *The New Experience of Childbirth*.[4]

The whole experience was astonishing. The only thing that compares with having your first baby is having your first book!

Since then I have written 35 more books, many published in other countries and languages, and revised and updated over the years. My *Good Birth Guides* for example, took the lid off hospitals.[5,6] It was a shock to some professionals that anyone should dare to publish a hospital guide like a hotel or restaurant directory. They denounced it as 'unscientific'. Of course it was. So is a hotel guide. But it gives the reader a basis on which to find out more and to compare what she wants with what women tell her about their experiences. After it came out some hospital administrators and obstetricians – only a handful, but it was a radical change – wrote to tell me what they were doing to improve things. Maternity hospitals have now become open to public audit.

My books celebrate the sexuality of birth and, I hope, can help women discover it for themselves. Articles regularly appear in the press (mostly women's and parenting magazines) about sex, pregnancy and motherhood, but in the form of either 'Let's get sexy again' or 'Sound medical information and advice'.

I explore the complexity and depth of female sexuality. Sex and birth are intimately connected with our sense of self-worth, joy in the power of our bodies, and freedom to express ourselves through them.

'I . . . never made the obvious connection between sexual feelings and birth until I witnessed a laboring woman whose husband was sitting at her side pull him closer and passionately kiss him during a long contraction. Her relaxation during this intense part of labor was instant and impressive. . . . The ecstatic and beautiful birth that resulted from this woman's pulling her husband to her for a kiss . . . enlarged my growing collection of practical techniques to pass along . . .'

Ina May Gaskin
Birth Matters[7]

1

DE-SEXING BIRTH

If you have had a painful labour or one which was distressing because you felt trapped (even if it was not particularly painful), you may think that sexual excitement and feelings during birth have no connection with each other. The sensations of labour obviously have nothing to do with being sexually titillated. Yet in a strange way the energy flowing through the body in childbirth, the pressure of contracting muscles, the downward movement of the baby and fanning open of soft tissues, can be powerfully erotic.

Some women compare birth with orgasm. One says, 'It's like having a baby. You build up to a climax. Then you push the baby's head out. It's the most wonderful feeling in the world ... the end feeling is the same.' Another woman tells me that the release she feels with orgasm is like that when her waters broke as she gave birth to her son.

Pain and pleasure are often very similar. Orgasm can bring a bitter-sweet pain: 'Orgasm is like a pain, a sweet pain that gets bigger and bigger and fills you up. Then as it ebbs you are left feeling content and throbbing.' One woman tells me that it is 'sensuous bordering on painful', and another, 'Sometimes the pleasure is so acute it is almost too much to bear, almost painful.' For many women there is a narrow, almost razor-edged separation, between intense pleasure and pain. Orgasm is a paradox: 'A painless pain, an ecstatic agony, a paralysed movement.' When women talk about orgasm they nearly always introduce the idea of 'tension increasing to explosion' which is followed by relaxation and a feeling of tiredness and heaviness. It is like 'bursting balloons', 'exploding bombs' or 'erupting volcanoes'. Time and time again they introduce images of waves crashing on the beach.

Orgasm is also essentially a giving and a flowing, 'like squeezing juice from a lemon'. For some it is a rhythmic blossoming: 'A flower opening'. For some it is movement, achievement and bliss: 'Like dancing on a sort of spring – getting higher, slipping back a bit – getting higher still and back a bit, and so on until you reach the top – the sort of explosive release which comes – like a broken honey pot with honey spreading through your body. It's lovely!'

For some women there is danger in these intense feelings: 'An orgasm builds slowly and bubbles before it finally explodes, then returns to a simmer once again. I would describe it as a kettle boiling.' One says, for example, that it is: 'A high build-up of electric power. When you have an orgasm it is like just before the fuse blows.' And there is a sense of urgency, having to put something right, 'like the car screaming out for someone to change gear'. Orgasm may be associated with an increasing sense of constriction – mounting anxiety, being lost or blinded – and then an overwhelming sense of relief – a fall into freedom. Another woman expresses this constriction followed by release when she says that, for her, orgasm is 'like a train going through a tunnel and suddenly emerging into bright daylight'.

Debra Pascali-Bonaro, an American birth educator, made a film called *Orgasmic Birth*. She said of her own birth-giving, 'It was the most overwhelming pleasure I have ever felt in my life.'[8]

In the second stage of labour each contraction can bring a series of orgasms as each one climaxes in pushing and release, mounts again, culminates in another, and so on. Unlike the male orgasm, which is usually a single tide of release, after which a man loses his erection, women have a multiple orgasm. It is the same with giving birth. Every contraction brings (for a while at least) waves of desire, climaxing in fulfilment when a woman's breathing speeds up and her breath is held voluntarily. This may happen two, three, four times – perhaps more – with each second stage contraction. It is the right time, and the only time, to push.

Women who have not experienced waves of orgasm – longing and climax – may think that references to orgasm are about the birth as the baby slides out. This is how it is for some women who have had an ecstatic birth, but a more general analogy is a multiple orgasm that comes in great rushes with each longing to push.

We are told that sex is different from childbirth. In the same way, it is considered indecent to experience intense physical satisfaction from breastfeeding. I understand why many people are embarrassed by the idea and believe that if a woman enjoys the rushes of the second stage she must be a sadomasochist. The important thing is that the orgasm is a side-effect, not the goal. We don't want mothers or midwives feeling that they have failed if the woman doesn't have an orgasm. There is already enough pressure on women to achieve the perfect birth these days, so adding orgasm to the wish list is a pretty tall order. And I would say to all the men out there, 'Please don't expect your partner to produce an orgasm. She may be faking it in bed, but don't expect her to fake it in childbirth.'

The Rhythm of Labour

The locus of many of the sensations felt in labour is an area about the size of your hand, deep in the pelvis. If you rest a hand above your pubis you will find the right place. The cervix opens beneath this area and much of the pain felt comes from it as it opens and is pulled up and over the baby's head. It may feel like a glowing fire which bursts into flames as a contraction builds up. Pain spreads from the cervix round into the small of the back until you are held in a tight grip from front to back for half a minute or so, after which it fades away again. This tightening is not haphazard. It is firm, regular, rhythmic. A woman who is enjoying her labour swings into the rhythm of contractions and her birth-giving may stimulate her to break into a powerful dance, her uterus creating the beat. She watches for it, concentrates on it, like an orchestra following the conductor.

It has been tempting for me to act this belly dance on demonstration marches if the police have urged us to 'keep moving'. It happened in 1990 when we were demonstrating in Vancouver for the re-creation of midwifery in Canada, for example. I welcomed police instructions and with my realistic baby doll and foam rubber vagina danced my way in front of the College of Medicine giving birth.

The sensations a woman experiences are at their most powerful in her sexual organs. Feelings of intense excitement pour through her genitals. In antenatal classes you may never learn this, or, because medical language obscures what we really feel, it may never be put into words which enable you to anticipate any powerful sexual sensation. The uterus, the vagina, the muscles enfolding the vagina and rectum, the lower back, the rectum and the anus, the buttocks, tissues around and between the vagina and anus, and the clitoris are all suffused with heat as if with liquid fire and pouring with radiant colour. It can be the most intensely sexual feeling a woman ever experiences, as strong as orgasm, even more compelling than orgasm. Some women find this sexuality disturbing because they feel out of control as the energy floods through them and they can do nothing to prevent it.

The Place of Birth

Michel Odent believes that women should give birth in the place they make love. Marsden Wagner, former Director of Women's and Children's Health in Europe for the World Health Organisation, says in Debra Pascali-Bonaro's film: 'It's got to be how it is when you make love with someone. It's got to be safe, secure and uninterrupted.'

The sexuality of natural birth stands in startling contrast to the institutional setting usually provided for the experience. It is as if we had to make love, pouring ourselves, body and mind, into the full expression of feeling, on a busy airport concourse, or in a gymnasium. Birth is usually treated as a medico-surgical crisis.

Women are fed into the hospital system at one end, are processed through it, and come out at the other with a baby. Instead of being a personal, private, intimate experience, the mother is on an assembly line. Even the way she sits or lies is dictated by the position of electrodes and catheters attached to her body and tubes tethering her to machines. And though professionals may be kind, labour becomes an ordeal because she is imprisoned in a situation outside her control.

'We need to restrain your hands otherwise you might contaminate *my* sterile field', the obstetrician explains, as the obstetric nurse or midwife puts the wrist straps onto the labouring woman. Her legs are raised and parted wide in lithotomy stirrups so that he has easy access to the perineum.

Now come the drapes, enveloping the lower half of the patient, including her feet, with a hole over the vagina for the baby to come through. The woman is effectively split into two halves, the lower end the 'working part', which is the property of the obstetrician, and the upper segment, consisting of head, neck, shoulders, breasts and arms, which, one suspects, the technician working down the other end would do away with if it were feasible.

In the position of a beetle on its back she is instructed to push the baby out.

One of the most pronounced differences between birth films in England and those in the USA is that in contemporary English ones the baby emerges from a hole in the woman's body which is seen to gradually open up, stretch wide, and give birth, whereas in American versions the baby often emerges through a hole in a sheet, and the woman who is bearing the child seems a long way from what is going on.

In England the tradition of midwifery means that the woman can co-operate as an active partner in the birth process, in any position in which she is most comfortable, and it is assumed that when she bears down she would prefer her head and shoulders to be well raised, rather than flat on a delivery table. Because almost invariably obstetricians do deliveries in the USA women are expected to submit as they might to a surgical operation. The lithotomy position rather than midwives is employed as routine in all deliveries and the woman is expected to push uphill without the force of gravity to help her and the baby give birth.

Even with a fairly sophisticated audience – one in Harvard – I realised that in showing an English birth film in which the woman's hands are not manacled and her whole perineum and vulva are put on view I was submitting them to a shocking experience. For above all in America the body is de-personalised. It is an object on a delivery table, and if, as in some films designed to show how good birth can be, the mother displays delight at delivery, the expression on her face takes place at the other end of the great divide between the birth-giving body swathed in sterile hospital garments and the head end where there is a person who feels emotion.

Women who have discovered that birth is a passionate sexual experience are likely to have given birth in their own homes or in birth units where there is unusual flexibility to enable them to behave without inhibition. In some hospitals and in birth rooms within them, a woman can have her baby without unnecessary intervention, in an atmosphere of peace and close intimacy, with helpers who have become her friends. She can explore the possibilities making a list of her priorities. The sexuality of birth is for the first time being experienced by women who are less concerned to remember all their breathing and relaxation exercises learned in antenatal classes, than to get in tune with their bodies and allow the energy of labour to flow through them. Even ten years ago a woman who cried out or grunted or groaned in labour often thought that she had 'failed'. She was anxious to 'keep control'. This stemmed from the teaching of 'psychoprophylaxis' which introduced a military-style discipline into preparation for childbirth and emphasised raising the pain threshold by keeping alert and using distraction techniques under the direction of a labour 'coach'. It is not surprising that women inculcated with such teachings, though they did well in labour and had a tremendous sense of triumph at delivery, were unlikely to experience childbirth as a psychosexual process.

It was very different for Elizabeth Davis, a midwife, who wrote of her own birth: 'For me, the ecstasy of the second stage occurred when my uterus and I were working as one, beyond signal and response. In this mode, a woman can literally deliver her own baby, sensing exactly when she can take more stretch and when to ease up, effortlessly breathing her baby out. . . . Later, my midwives said they wished they had the birth on tape, it was so perfectly controlled. But 'controlled' is not the way I would describe my process, as I wasn't really holding back. Beyond attunement, there was union, perfect union.'[9]

Elizabeth Davis discussed the relations between sexuality and bonding, too. Sexual hormones play an important part in behaviour immediately following birth. Research conducted with sheep has shown that when non-pregnant sheep are given oestrogen and progestogen and stimulated vaginally they react to newborn lambs as if they were their mothers. Newly delivered ewes accept lambs that are not their own. Sheep whose pelvic floors are anaesthetised during labour, however, are likely to reject their newborns in the first half-hour post-partum.[10,11]

Many procedures that are an accepted part of childbirth today, and which make it difficult for a woman to discover anything sexual in labour, have been introduced to formalise the relations between professionals and patients and to repress and inhibit any expression of emotion. These practices are part of the hospital institution, sanctified in the form of unquestioned routines that are justified on the grounds that they are for the safety of the baby, even when no research has been done to examine these claims.

Barbara Katz Rothman described the second stage of her labour: 'I felt myself opening, felt the head push through, a beautiful total sense of openness . . .'[12]

Speaking to the conference of the 1992 Midwives' Alliance of North America she said:

'The history of Western obstetrics is the history of technologies of separation. We've separated milk from breasts, mothers from babies, fetuses from pregnancies, sexuality from procreation, pregnancy from motherhood. And finally we're left with the image of the fetus as a free-floating being alone, analogous to man in space, with the umbilical cord tethering the placental ship, and the mother reduced to the empty space that surrounds it.'[13]

Even if a pregnant woman came to feel that birth could be sexual and sought to let her body come alive in labour in the same way as it does in passionate lovemaking, she would usually find that she was up against so many obstacles in hospitals that it was easier just to give in and let the professionals take over. There are very few institutions in which a woman can feel free to be herself, allow emotions to sweep through her and do whatever she wants to do. She becomes, in effect, an object on which doctors act.

Images of Birth

Women have depicted birth and the life-giving power of female sexuality in richly varied ways long before the start of recorded history. The earliest known portrayals are the ancient fertility goddess, and these images have survived the centuries and are still to be found in traditional cultures in Mexico, Peru and other South American countries today. This goddess also appeared as a geometric shape, the hooked diamond, often with a cross inside the diamond to represent the child, as in Turkish kelims. The shape persists in women's weaving and other artefacts made by women in many countries all over the world, including North Africa, India, Thailand and the islands of Oceania. It is the birth symbol, usually unknown to men.

Another symbol is the teardrop familiar in Paisley designs which represents the tree of life and dates from the Babylonian era. This fertility symbol originally depicted a curled palm frond. The motif passed into Celtic art and, probably in the seventeenth century, to Kashmir where it was woven into shawls.

When I asked carpet dealers in Morocco, all male, to explain to me the meaning of the hooked diamond in carpets woven by women they suggested 'men at prayer', 'a two-humped camel' and 'a mosque'. They saw these shapes with men's eyes. It is not only in North Africa that men and women have a different way of seeing. We are surrounded by images which can be different depending on whether men or women are looking at them – in kitchens, shops, on TV and in hospitals.

Open any obstetric textbook and there are illustrations of headless torsos, legs splayed and amputated, perineums bulging, with forceps blades inserted, arrows indicating the correct outward and upward pull. Generations of medical students have been taught with images like these to see women's bodies as de-personalised, fragmented and sexless. They have been trained to perceive the female body as posing a mechanical dilemma. Birth is primarily a matter of engineering.

In one photograph of what appears to be a woman's trunk the body might as well be that of a corpse, heavily draped so that no flesh is visible. There is a hole in the sheet through which the fetus is to be ejected. This is an obstetrician's view of a woman's body.

A dramatic photograph of a breech delivery shows a band of gowned and masked priest-like figures lit by a white light, cold and hard as ice. The woman is not visible. There is only that startling white, those ceremonial figures – and darkness. The drama is in what the obstetrician and his acolytes are doing. The woman might as well not exist.

Today artists have reclaimed the creative force and flowing energy of childbirth and are producing vivid images that are woman-centred, which focus on the welling-up of power, the strength of the mother, the unfurling petals of flesh, and the sense of incarnation deep in every birth. Some of these artists are men who have shared in birth and are astonished by and in awe of it. Most are women who strive to stress the oneness with nature, the irresistible power of creation and sexual ecstasy. One of the most compelling of these is by an Inuit sculptor, who has done a whole series on birth, and in my collection of birth sculptures from all over the world I treasure a soapstone carving by her of a woman giving birth with the strength of mountains, thighs spread wide. It is a celebration of sexuality.

Images of birth which celebrate the energy of women's bodies, as these do, could be on the walls of every medical student's classroom and every hospital. They would provide an antidote to the medical way of viewing the pelvis and perineum as detached from a woman.

It is one way in which those who are striving for woman-centred care might reach the minds of medical students and obstetricians, and even, perhaps, start to change the way they think about birth so that they can acknowledge it as a psychosexual experience.

The Depersonalisation of Birth

The Victorian doctor's role was that of guardian with ward, father with child, teacher with pupil and father confessor with supplicant.

In the late nineteenth century there was much discussion among doctors about how to remove the sexuality from pelvic examinations.[14] Should the doctor look away from his female patient while doing a vaginal examination or stare with concentration at her face so that she could be sure that he was not looking at her genitals? Should a female chaperone always be present? The gynaecologist had to rely upon 'the touch' and must never reveal the patient's genitals. In the training of doctors the emphasis was put on rituals to maintain a woman's modesty.

Childbirth became increasingly mechanised after the Second World War. Doctors came back from the armed forces and wanted to rebuild their interrupted careers. They replaced midwives, and new teams were set up in which midwives were subordinate members, taking their orders from doctors who were eager to use the organisational skills they had acquired on land, sea and in the air as they worked in battle. They wanted to make childbirth more efficient, and save babies' lives. The fetus became the patient who they saved and its survival depended on them committing themselves to disciplining the maternal body. To do this birth had to be de-sexed.

The obstetrician-as-scientist came on the scene in the second half of the twentieth century, when women started to give birth in hospitals.

The obstetrician is on his own territory in a maternity hospital. He has the power, technological equipment and supporting staff to turn every birth into a medico-surgical procedure. This is the case whether the doctor is male or female. It enables a woman's body to be treated as if it were separate from herself as a person. Each woman is treated as an ambulant pelvis during pregnancy and a contracting uterus in labour. It is assumed that doctors know what is best for a patient better than she can know herself.

Once hospital birth became the norm, more and more women gave birth on narrow, hard delivery tables under bright lights with their legs raised and fixed wide apart in lithotomy stirrups. Doctors and nurses wore sterile garments, gowns, caps, overshoes, masks and surgical gloves. The upper and lower ends of the patient's torso were divided by drapes, the isolated lower section designated as the obstetrician's 'sterile field', which was out of bounds to the mother herself, and only he could touch. This was always a fiction, because the proximity of the vagina to the anus means that it cannot really be sterile.

In the 1950s and 1960s women often laboured for long periods alone, without their partners or other family members. What had been a personal, intimate and passionate act of creating life, often became a process in which a woman was treated with cool, brisk efficiency or was left to 'get on with it' until the obstetrician put in an appearance, anaesthetised her, applied forceps and pulled the baby out like a rabbit from a hat. The Medical Defence Union Consent to Treatment stated:

> 'The Union does not consider that a maternity patient need give her written consent to any operation or manipulative procedures . . . When she enters hospital for her confinement it can be assumed that she assents to any necessary procedures, including the administration of a local, general or other anaesthetic.'[15]

The obstetric delivery is a caricature of normal childbirth. Not only were the woman's legs suspended in stirrups but her wrists, too, were often bound. Her body became the passive object on which the doctor acted to effect delivery. She lay flat on her back while he got on with the job at the lower end of her body. Her perineum was shaved as bald as an egg and the medical view of her was of a heavily draped, lumpy object, like a sofa shrouded in dust covers, and a central window in the cloth with an opening in which the ball-shaped mass of the fetal head could be seen descending through the smooth, shiny, bulging balloon of the perineum. It appeared that the doctor was no longer doing things to a woman's body, but was servicing a reproductive machine.

A Package Deal

Another theme in the relationship between obstetrician and patient which runs parallel with the emergence of doctor-as-scientist was that of the deliverer with the power to prescribe drugs to take away pain, who promises the woman, 'Trust me, do what I say and you need not suffer'.

There is a price to pay for such solicitude. Anaesthesia makes more intervention possible. And because it interferes with a woman's normal physiological functions and usually also affects the fetus, it makes this intervention more likely. As a result, women may be offered a package deal of pain relief plus forceps lift-out and whatever else may be necessary – intravenous uterine stimulants, a catheter to drain urine, a surgical cut to open the vagina and insert stitches in it afterwards, pain-relieving drugs and sleeping pills in the week after delivery, and so on.

It started in the United States in the 1920s with Joseph DeLee's system of 'prophylactic forceps'. This entailed sedation, an episiotomy (the cut) and the introduction of forceps to pull the baby's head out over the perineum. Since this method made delivery much more painful, general anaesthesia was used in the second stage of labour, and the woman would wake up to learn that she had a baby. A mix of mood-changing, pain-relieving and sleep-inducing drugs was used for the earlier part of labour. One of the most notorious of these, scopolamine, was widely employed and is still in use in many hospitals in the USA. It makes the woman confused and restless, often so much out of her mind that she has to be nursed in a high-barred and padded crib or wear a kind of straitjacket or football helmet in case she injures herself. From the delivery room she goes straight to the 'recovery room', where there is another set of equipment to resuscitate her if necessary.

To increase efficiency, birth is a production-line operation. Tasks are divided between different professionals. A woman being processed through labour is admitted by one member of the staff, supervised in the first stage by others, delivered by yet another group and cared for subsequently by a different post-partum team. Often she has never met any of these people before. It is task-centred rather than woman-centred care, and, especially for the poorest and the least educated, takes place in an alien environment among total strangers, without explanation, regardless of a woman's own wishes and feelings, and without anyone there who can understand what she is going through.

It was not until the beginning of the 1970s that it became acceptable practice in most UK hospitals for the baby's father or another close family member to be present during labour and delivery. The battle for one of the most natural rights is still being fought in some American hospitals.

The Spontaneous Second Stage

As full dilatation of the cervix is reached there is often a pause in spontaneous birthing. I call it the 'rest and be thankful' phase. It is a time when a woman can recoup her strength and relax completely before the rush of energy that comes with the action of the second stage. Unfortunately this is often when midwives get anxious about lack of progress, urge the woman to push even though she has no passionate drive to do so, and intervene by pressing down on the uterus or taking deep breaths that the mother is instructed to imitate. Instead, everyone should all drop shoulders, relax and *wait*.

When a woman is helped to do whatever she feels like doing in the second stage, adopting positions, moving and breathing in any way she wants to, the second stage can become an intense sexual experience. Rhythms are unforced, and she is not striving to reach what appears an unattainable goal or put on a performance, but listens to and trusts her body. She pushes only when the desire is urgent and overwhelming. She feels extraordinary and intensely sexual sensations as the baby's head presses first against her anus and then down through the concertina-like folds of her vagina until it feels like a hard bud in the middle of a great, open peony. Perhaps she puts her fingers down to feel the hard top of the baby's head as it presses through spreading tissues. She is in touch with what is happening. There is no need to use counter-pressure against the baby's head, to tell her to pant, to rotate the head externally or to do any of the other manipulations which are often necessary when guiding a desperate woman, and which have become part of the routines of delivery.

Her face lights up as she realises that this is her baby being born, a living being from her body, and she can see its head and reach down and feel it as it slides into life. Suddenly she is full, stretched to her utmost, as if she is a seed pod bursting. There is a moment of waiting, of awe, of the kind of tension which occurs just before orgasm, and then suddenly the baby passes through, the whole body slips out in a rush of warm flesh, a fountain of water, a peak of overwhelming surprise and the little body is against her skin, kicking against her thighs or swimming up over her belly. She reaches out to hold her baby, firm, solid, with bright, bright eyes. A peak sexual experience, the birth passion, becomes the welcoming of a new person into life. All the intense sexual feelings of labour and delivery have culminated in the passion, hunger and fulfilment of a mother and her newborn baby.

Ina May Gaskin, who created a new style of midwifery at The Farm in Tennessee, rediscovering the kind of care that was part of traditional, non-professional midwifery, has said that 20 per cent of women she attended in labour experienced orgasm.[16]

A lawyer in Brighton, aged 31, who experienced an orgasmic birth wrote:

'I am well aware how many women reading this will open their eyes wide in disbelief and dismiss my experience as some sort of exhaustion-induced fantasy. Before it happened to me, I would probably have done the same. Confessing to my friends, who have, in most cases, experienced agonising 10- or 20-hour labours, that mine was the most enjoyable seven hours of my life has been tough enough. But when I add that it was accompanied by an orgasm, I find myself being made to feel in some way strange or deluded. It's better to keep the whole experience to myself . . . It was the most incredible feeling that began in my pelvis and rippled through my entire lower body. It was wave upon wave of what can only be described as pure pleasure . . . After the birth, I was so excited that I wanted to share what had happened with friends, but their reactions quickly taught me that this was probably something that I should think of as my own private but wonderful experience and keep it to myself.'[17]

Because a woman has been able to give birth spontaneously, she acts spontaneously after the baby is born, too. There is a flow of feeling which opens her arms to cradle her child, and causes blood to rush to warm her breasts and make her nipples firm so that she is ready and eager when the baby starts to seek her breast, latches on and presses out the rich colostrum.

Anyone who, far from experiencing orgasmic birth, found it a painful ordeal, has not failed to be a 'real mother'. If you are to know the thrill of childbirth and then spontaneously nurture your baby, you need to be nurtured, too. You are not just a baby-producing apparatus, but a woman who should be cherished in an environment where pregnancy and birth are regarded as personal and intimate experiences, and you can trust your body and express yourself through it. You are acknowledged as an adult, taking on responsibility for a new life, not a passive patient undergoing a medico-surgical crisis.

Western society generally fails to provide such an environment, and medical and nursing routines impose a ceremonial order, reducing the mother to the status of a child, and de-sexing her. Care in childbirth must change radically if women are to enjoy the power liberated in their bodies, to bond naturally with their babies, and go on to handle the major challenges of motherhood.

Sex, birth and motherhood are not really different, conflicting experiences. They are part of a continuum. What we learn from each deepens our understanding of other aspects of our lives.

2

GENITAL GEOGRAPHY

The vagina, the shape formed by the lips of the vagina, and the size and form of the clitoris are different in different women, just as our faces are different. There is no one 'right' way to be.

We can explore our genital organs with a finger and look at them in a mirror, too. We examine our faces in a mirror almost every day – sometimes several times a day. Think of the amount of time a woman spends staring at the reflection of her face, but how little she spends getting to know her genitals by touch and sight.

So when you have some quiet time alone, sit comfortably with a mirror and small table lamp or torch, and take an opportunity to understand how you are constructed, the configuration of flesh folds and the relationship between different organs and their relative sizes. You can then explore the feelings you get when you touch different parts of the genitals.

What You Can See and Touch

The curved sloping front, which in some women is bushy and in others only lightly covered, is sometimes called the 'mound of Venus'. Hair may spread quite a long way up your abdomen and down the insides of your legs, too. In some cultures – Russia for example – women shave off all pubic hair. This is becoming increasingly fashionable in Western countries now. The only hair that remains is on a woman's head.

At the base of the curve of the mound of Venus and tucked behind it, feel the hard ridge of the pubic bone that forms the front of the pelvis. Move your hand down between your legs and you reach the hair-covered outer lips or labia, like the thick, fleshly lips of a tropical flower. They do not look neat and tidy like the diagrams in anatomy books.

If you part the lips you come to another set of lips inside. These are thinner, smooth and silky, and glisten with moisture, especially when you are sexually aroused. Look closely and you can see through the outer tissues a network of veins. The inner lips often curve out and over the outer lips so that there is a light shaded strip projecting from within the outer labia, a bit like a conch shell.

Like our mouths, these lips do not form a standard cupid-bow shape. These curved and convoluted petal shapes often occur in orchids and other flowers. Confronting them in a mirror they may look very 'primitive', compared to the regularity we superimpose on our cosmetically decorated faces. You may even think they are ugly. Perhaps it is significant that a woman sometimes spends a long time making up her mouth with lip-liner and lipstick, hoping to make it conform to an ideal and regular shape. Some women have cosmetic surgery to tidy up their genitals.

Notice the colours of the outer and inner lips – violet, dusky pink, crimson, tawny brown, gold and blue. The outer lips are darker than the inner ones. They may be a deep brown or black, whereas the inner lips are pink or red. In pregnancy an added blood supply to the pelvic area makes these colours more dramatic, and the red shades brighten. After the baby is born they change again and there is more blue.

The Hymen

In childhood the hymen, a fine layer of tissue, closes the entrance to the vagina partially or completely. In some women this is strong and resistant and makes intercourse difficult. Occasionally it even needs to be cut under local anaesthetic. Usually the hymen is torn easily when a tampon is first inserted, if a woman slides her own finger in, or sometimes as a result of sports that put the area under stress. There may be slight spotting of blood when this occurs. Most women probably do not notice when the hymen is first torn, and there is no reason why it should be painful. If you look closely you may still see the frilled edges of the remaining hymen. The presence or absence of a hymen is nothing to do with being a virgin. Though the exhibition of a blood-stained sheet following defloration on the marriage night forms a part of wedding ceremonies in some peasant communities in the Mediterranean, this is a purely ritual act and does not reflect physiological reality. To get the blood a chicken is often slaughtered.

The Clitoris

The exquisitely sensitive clitoris lies at the upper end of the vagina between the folds of the labia with its smooth, curved tip, the glans, projecting like a pea, a little like the pink eraser stuck on the end of a pencil. There is often quite a thick fold of skin like a hood or wimple over the clitoris and you may not be able to see it until you part the inside lips with your fingers.

Many women who have never before explored the clitoris might think that men, at any rate, would have a fairly good idea what it looks like. But Shere Hite in her *Report on Male Sexuality*, wrote that most men learned about the clitoris from books and their idea of it is derived from illustrations encountered in sex manuals or biology textbooks. When they did describe it, however, those who had actually seen one produced some vivid and often tender descriptions: 'a small nipple', 'a pearly little head', 'a tiny titty jelly bean', 'a red pea coming out of its shell', 'like a baby clam – very ripe and inviting', 'a small leaf', 'a cross between a small shrimp and a small appendage with an excitable tip', and even 'like an ice cream cone in a raging storm'.[18]

Slip your finger down a little further to the entrance of the vagina, and press inward. Then you can feel the root of the clitoris lying beneath the glans. When you squeeze it repeatedly you will notice that the glans plumps up in response to the stimulation.

Slide your finger in further still, pressing forward and there is a pad of thick, spongy tissue between your pubic bone and the urethra. Then press down and you will discover another pad of thick, spongy tissue between the vagina and the anus. These spongy tissues surrounding the vagina protect it and when you are sexually excited become engorged and thicker still.

The Cervix

Kneel and slip your finger deeper inside your vagina and you may be able to feel the lowest part of your uterus, the cervix. If you have not yet had a baby it feels like the tip of your nose, except if you are ovulating, when it gets softer. If you have had a baby it feels more like a chin with a deep dimple, and when you are ovulating the dimple may feel like a soft, relaxed mouth.

This dimple is a small hole or slit in the centre of the cervix, and is called the os. With ovulation, the os opens and mucus from the cervix bathes the vagina, keeping it clean and slightly acid. The mucus is usually white but changes so that when a ripe ovum is waiting to be fertilised it is of a clear slippery consistency. This encourages the movement of sperm up into the fallopian tubes where fertilisation takes place. The mucus increases until the day before you ovulate you feel really damp. After ovulation the mucus decreases. You have least mucus during a period and feel driest immediately after it is over.

Some women use a speculum to examine their cervix to get to know how it looks when it is healthy and at different times in the menstrual cycle. If you want to do this buy one so that you can examine yourself. Try to get hold of the plastic type. Metal is not good. Plastic is much easier, lighter and more comfortable to use, and costs less. It is a kind of 'beak' which you insert into your vagina. Once it is inside open it and the two halves separate the walls of your vagina. Use a mirror, and if you have a torch shine it onto the mirror, not onto the cervix, to get the best view.

You cannot feel the main part of your uterus. It is shaped like a pear or fig, with the stalk end tilted down into your vagina. Sometimes this 'stalk' is tilted forwards, sometimes backwards. It is sometimes said that a backwards-tilted uterus makes it more difficult to conceive, but this is not so.

The uterus is an active, contracting organ from the first menstrual period until the menopause or after. It is not just a bag hanging there, but a living network of muscle fibres which, though not under conscious control, tighten and release regularly in response to stimuli at different times in the menstrual cycle. The cramps often felt during a period are simply tightenings of the uterus. When you have an orgasm your uterus contracts too. Sometimes it goes on contracting after the orgasm, and occasionally this can produce abdominal cramp. During pregnancy it contracts regularly in rehearsal for the birth. It also contracts when the breasts, in particularly the nipples, are stimulated. There is a connection between the uterus and the nipples, and a woman who has breastfed knows that when a baby is sucking steadily in the first few days after birth it is almost as if the mouth was pulling on an invisible string in the uterus, producing 'after-pains'. These contractions tone the uterus so that it returns to its previous shape and size.

Pelvic Floor Muscles

Put your fingers inside your vagina and squeeze the muscles around it, about half-way up inside. If you are not quite sure whether you have located them, squeeze as if you want to prevent urine flowing. Those you can feel with your fingers are the ones nearest the outside.

During orgasm they contract at 0.8 second intervals, pressing on the clitoris, the vaginal tissues and the inner layers of muscles supporting the bladder and uterus. You can also tighten the muscles deliberately in a steady rhythm to increase sexual arousal.

The pelvic floor muscles form a figure of eight around the vagina and anus. They support everything in the bony pelvic girdle and, at one remove, everything in your abdominal cavity. They are probably the most important muscles in a woman's body. The biggest muscle, the pubococcygeus, sweeps across from the bone forming the front of the pelvis to the one at the very bottom of the spine. There are layers of muscles, like coiled springs, surrounding the urethra – the tube leading from the bladder – as well as the vagina and the anus.

A rich network of blood vessels criss-crosses the outside of the vagina, the uterus, fallopian tubes and ovaries. Increased or reduced blood flow to these organs also results in a change in their shape and size.

Bringing the Pelvic Floor Alive

The tone and vitality of the pelvic floor muscles are very important for a woman's sex life. If they are slack and she does not know how to use them, she is missing out on a whole aspect of experience – involving the deep layers of muscle that surround the vagina and rectum and press against her uterus and bladder.

To discover whether your pelvic floor muscles are strong interrupt a stream of urine and see if you can stop it completely. Then let urine flow again. Now interrupt it again – and so on. If you can do this then they are in good condition. Even so, we can go on from there to learn how to use them more actively. There are ways of exercising these muscles to give added pleasure in sex and to delight a partner.

The first movement is simple – it is the vaginal kiss. Think of the ring of muscle fibres about half way up inside your vagina and tighten it. The O shape will change to a smaller almond shape. Hold it a few seconds and then release. We do this spontaneously when making love. During orgasm this movement occurs at split-second intervals as a sequence of rapid vaginal kisses.

Now imagine a small, soft fruit – the size of a cherry – inside the circle of muscles and use them as if you were chewing and eating the fruit. You will probably find that you are using the muscles of your mouth, too. Then 'swallow' the fruit with a smooth movement as if you were drawing it into your uterus. Rest a few seconds and now 'eat' another piece of fruit. And rest again. This may be quite tiring at first, so allow for regular rest times.

Now imagine a much larger soft fruit – a peach or apricot – with a smooth, velvety skin. With your pelvic floor muscles, 'scan' the curved surface of this imaginary fruit in a sweeping, stroking movement. It is a much slower, larger movement than in the previous exercise.

Now imagine that the fruit is crushed and juice is flowing from it. Slowly suck in the juice with your muscles. Again you may discover that you are making similar movements with your lips, mouth and throat. Now rest.

As you have been doing this you will have realised that you were contracting not only the muscles of the vagina but those which encircle the rectum, anus and urethra, too. This is normal because the muscle fibres are all interconnected, so that when you firmly contract any part of the pelvic floor other parts contract as well.

When a muscle is not strong enough to cope with a sustained contraction it starts to tremble. This may have happened to you with some of the longer, firmer contractions. It is why it is a good idea, if your muscles are not well toned to start with, to practise light, short movements and build up activity gradually. When a muscle is contracted hard the flow of blood through it is reduced, and hence its oxygen. When it is released the blood flows through faster. So when you contract and release in a dance-like movement you increase the oxygen supply to the muscle and avoid straining it.

In lovemaking other muscles work together with the pelvic floor and get caught up in the same interplay of movement. Muscles connected with our breathing are affected, too, so that when we contract and release the pelvic floor we are probably also catching our breath in little gasps. We may spontaneously squeeze our thighs or press our buttocks together. This has the effect of further gripping a partner's hand or penis.

If we are very excited pelvic floor movements spread to whole body movements. The pelvis rocks forwards and backwards. When the pelvic floor is contracted we tend to rock the pelvis forward, press down the small of the back and flatten the abdominal muscles. When the pelvic floor muscles are released the lower back hollows slightly and the abdominal muscles relax.

Lie on your back with your knees drawn up and feet flat on the floor. Tighten your pelvic floor muscles, press your buttocks together and press the small of your back against the floor. Then release your pelvic floor and the muscles of the lower back and abdomen. Let the tightening and release flow right through the whole pelvic area. Do this about ten times.

You may have noticed that other muscles get involved in the movement, too: shoulders, hands, muscles for the face and feet, for example. Now let all these muscles join in the activity and *exaggerate* the movement. Contract the muscles of the pelvis and anything else you want to tighten. Then release and contract and release and contract, and continue doing this, letting the movement flow from the activity of the pelvic floor, which is the pacemaker. It is the start of a belly dance. Now relax completely for a few moments and think of the vagina as soft and warm.

This is one way of 'waking up' a pelvic floor that is not tuning us into sex.

The best all-round everyday exercise for toning pelvic floor muscles is the 'lift', as described in Chapter 11, Sex After the Baby Comes.

In childbirth as you are pushing your baby out let these muscles bulge forward. In this way you help the baby's presenting part – usually the head – descend and rotate into the best position for birth.

The structure of the female genital organs is like a theatre in which is enacted a dramatic cyclical pattern of change that starts from the time just before a woman's very first period and ends after menopause.

Many of these organs are constructed with a good deal of 'slack', like a very loose weave, pleated dress, and blood vessels, like rivers with hundreds of tributaries, etch a wide band surrounding them. They are pliable and can change their size and form. In response to thoughts and feelings the folds of convoluted tissue spread and open out so that the shape of the vagina changes. When we blush, feel self-conscious and turn red, our faces do not radically change their shape. An equivalent flow of blood to the vagina, however, leads to plumping up and opening, like a bud bursting into full flower.

Examining anatomic structures gives very little idea of the immense variations of which a woman's genital organs are capable. The entire process is one of ebb and flow, folding and unfolding, opening and closing. This happens not only in the parts where obvious changes can be felt with your fingers – the lips, the vagina and clitoris – but deep inside – in the uterus, the fallopian tubes and the ovaries.

3

SEX AND PREGNANCY

When It Is Difficult to Start a Baby

Sexual spontaneity disappears the moment you start being concerned that the baby you wanted is not coming and that you must have intercourse on special days of the month if you are going to conceive. Sex then becomes a means to an end.

It is bound to affect your feelings about lovemaking and then a whole range of other emotions: hope, frustration, irritation and despair, for *both* partners. If you are not certain when you ovulate, or even if you ovulate regularly, you have to take your temperature first thing in the morning, keep a chart, and perhaps also examine your mucus. Then the moment comes that intercourse is required but it turns out that he is away, is dead tired, or has flu. Or you have had a quarrel and the last thing you really feel like is making love. Intercourse under such circumstances becomes a duty which must be performed, proof that you want a baby enough to take the trouble, and a gamble in which you take your chances against an obstinate fate.

It can be more complicated than that. If you want to give a baby the best start in life you probably should be environmentally conscious. You will have had to give up smoking or drinking heavily, since that produces more inactive sperm. Very hot baths, and a man's tight underpants and jeans can also immobilise sperm. Potency and fertility are related to good nutrition. But perhaps your partner finds it very difficult to stop smoking, had to skip lunch, and dropped into a bar. The man may get to feel that he is being treated like a stud bull, allowed to have intercourse only when the time is right, and may be denied intercourse in the whole second half of the month when you might possibly be pregnant, because you are worried that he could dislodge a minuscule fertilised cell cluster. This puts stress on the relationship.

As soon as doctors get involved, trying to start a baby becomes a clinical exercise. It is almost as if the woman and the doctor become the procreating couple. You and your partner may be told to have intercourse within a specified time before you go to the doctor so that you arrive with semen in your vagina. The man may be required to go to the doctor's office to masturbate and produce a semen specimen to be examined under the microscope in order to reveal the ratio of live sperm. Healthy semen probably contains a minimum of twenty million sperm to each cubic centimetre. That test is often performed after a series of investigations have taken place on the woman, though it is one of the simpler and more obvious ones that should be carried out early in the process, since at least 20 per cent of cases of infertility show that the man is responsible.

A man sometimes feels that not only are his sperm being called into question, but his very masculinity. He is being pronounced inadequate. That may affect the way he makes love and his capacity to have and sustain an erection.

So a couple are both under stress and often in a state where the strain they feel finds an outlet in accusations against each other – perhaps he does not really care or genuinely want this baby – or they simply do not understand each other's feelings.

Anxiety about having intercourse at the time of ovulation, and avoiding it until that time comes, sometimes stops it altogether. A woman who was told that she must take her basal body temperature, abstain from intercourse for five days before her temperature went up, and then have intercourse promptly, discovered that her cycles became completely unpredictable, 20 days one month and 45 the next. The doctor suggested that the couple should not gear lovemaking to the temperature chart, but have intercourse whenever they felt like it. In two months she became pregnant.

Seeking help can often alleviate anxiety, however. Perhaps 20 per cent of women get pregnant between their first consultation with a specialist and the doctor initiating treatment. It may be because at last the couple have relaxed in the knowledge that they are doing something about it.

If you both know that you are likely to be under emotional pressure to start a baby you can help each other by talking openly about your feelings before they mount up to become a barrier between you. The process involved in trying to conceive that elusive baby could actually bring you closer together.

Lying close *after* intercourse is important, too. Ejaculation and receiving semen is not just an exercise to try to make a baby. A woman may have been told to lie in one position, on her back with a pillow under her bottom, for 20 or 30 minutes after intercourse, to give the sperm the best chance of travelling through the cervix, but she should not have to lie like that while her partner turns over and goes to sleep. It can be a time for loving and close tenderness. She may want further stimulation to have an orgasm during this time. Both of you need to know that you are loved and wanted for *yourselves*.

Nausea in Early Pregnancy

The nausea and vomiting common in the first three months is a sexual turn-off. Many women never experience it, but those who do may feel sick not only on waking in the morning but also in the early evening. For some it lasts right through the day.

Even if you feel rather better by bedtime, constant nausea makes it impossible to feel erotic. One woman, on what was supposed to be a romantic second honeymoon which coincided with the sixth and seventh weeks of her pregnancy, remembers the details of the toilet bowl in the hotel and the tiles and plumbing around it with much greater clarity than anything else about the holiday. Her husband lay in bed reading thrillers while she retched and vomited in the bathroom.

You may have nausea with one pregnancy, but not with another. Tiredness and 'overdoing things' often play a part in it. Eating regularly is important to avoid letting your stomach get empty. Small, frequent meals are better than large ones hours apart.

If you vomit you may be anxious about how this may be affecting the baby. 'I felt really awful,' one woman said. 'Drained of all vitality, smelly, with a tinny taste in my mouth. I wondered where this pregnancy radiance was. I felt ghastly! And sex was out of the question.'

Nausea often does not last after the first three months and you will probably wake up one morning feeling quite different or realise with surprise, as you get to the end of the day, that for the first time you have not felt sick.

At the end of pregnancy, when the baby's head engages it feels as if there is very little room for anything else and penetration is uncomfortable. Explore upright positions, side-lying and nestling with your partner behind. These give you freedom to move and take pressure off your bump.

Breasts

In the first weeks your breasts may feel very tender. Changes which make them ready for later feeding the baby, are some of the first obvious ways in which your body adapts to pregnancy. The little bumps around your nipples, called Montgomery's tubercles, get bigger and the breasts larger. A bra may feel uncomfortably tight and some women are so sensitive that they feel bruised. What is often called 'a good uplift bra' is necessary and even though this conjures up a picture of some monstrous contraption hoisting you into a different architectural shape, all it means is that there should be firm support *under* your breasts (around the midriff) and straps wide enough to take the extra pull of weight. Some women feel so uncomfortable in bed that they wake up with pressure against their breasts and prefer to wear a 'sleep' bra at night.

When this happens you cannot think of your breasts as erotic objects or playthings, even though a small-breasted woman may like them being larger and be proud of her new figure. A pregnant woman is very easily hurt by a lover who likes to pummel, bite or suck energetically, as some men do. Any nipple stimulation must be very gentle, and breast stroking should start with touch which is as light as a feather and only becomes firmer if it feels good.

In fact, this is one of the most obvious things about sex in pregnancy. A partner needs to be gentle at all times. Even if you enjoyed rough love-bites and a bit of sexual grappling before you were pregnant, you are most unlikely to now. It can feel as if you and your baby are under attack.

In a state of sexual arousal breasts swell by as much as 25 per cent. So when you get sexually excited you top up your already enlarged breasts as more blood rushes to the veins and tissues become further engorged. This is why, even when you are highly aroused, you may flinch when touched and then suddenly feel very much on the defensive.

Worrying about Miscarriage

Fear of miscarriage also has a marked effect on sexual feelings and on the capacity to be aroused in the first place. If you have already lost a baby in the first few months of a previous pregnancy, or have any bleeding at the beginning of this one, you may feel apprehensive and be almost 'holding on', both physically and emotionally, to this pregnancy. The result is that you see sex as a direct threat to the baby and are far too tense to relax and enjoy lovemaking. A woman who is anxious tends to lock her muscles in a state of contraction, not only those in her face which give her an anxious expression, but others all over her body. A man, too, may be very nervous and feel that he is a danger to the pregnancy, and a couple trigger further anxiety in each other. They may avoid cuddling and caressing because they are so fearful of sexual arousal.

The stress of worrying about miscarriage could increase

the chance of miscarriage. Little is known about the effects of stress on early pregnancy, but it is reasonable to assume that physiological changes which occur under acute stress – changes in the biochemistry of the blood, for example, and the way it flows through the blood vessels in the uterus – can affect the developing embryo.

Doctors usually advise against intercourse if a woman has any spotting of blood in the first 12 weeks or has miscarried in the previous pregnancy. Most women probably feel safer avoiding intercourse if they have any bleeding, though up to one-third of women in any antenatal class say that they have a slight bloodstained discharge somewhere around the time when the first or second period would have been due – and go on to have a normal pregnancy and a healthy baby. They often do not tell a doctor about this, who may not realise just how common it is.

A doctor who has advised against intercourse sometimes forgets to say: 'You are past the time when you are most likely to miscarry', and the couple continue not only to avoid sex, but often any form of lovemaking as well, right through pregnancy, or feel terribly guilty about it if they *do* make love. This is another way of medicalising pregnancy.

Miscarriage produces an imprint for the loss of self-confidence. This is likely to be massive after you have told other people that you are expecting a baby, and if you have already missed two or three periods and feel that the pregnancy is well established. It is bound to affect how you feel about sex and trusting your body.

It helps if you are prepared for what family members, friends, work colleagues, and even casual acquaintances, may say in an attempt to offer sympathy – things that leave you feeling worse than before.

'You should be glad you can conceive, anyway. Some women can't.' True, but another woman's misfortune can't make you any happier. And you are bound to wonder whether you can even conceive next time.

'*Well, you didn't start the baby on purpose did you? So it can't matter so much.*'
The way you felt when you first discovered you were pregnant may be quite different from your feelings a few weeks later, and it is certainly different from the emotional turmoil you are in now.

'*Isn't it lucky you miscarried so early? It would have been much worse later.*'
This is psychologically inept and infuriating.

'*Don't allow yourself to get upset. It's bad for your children/ husband/dog.*'
This makes you feel guiltier still. Why can't you control yourself? For the moment you are concerned with your own emotions, not theirs. You have a right to be upset.

'*Better luck next time!*'
Whoever says this would feel more comfortable if you smile and forget all about it, please. Your unhappiness is embarrassing. Actually, just now you are not sure you could face a 'next time'.

'*It was probably just as well. There must have been something wrong with the baby.*'
To be told you were producing a deformed baby does not make you more cheerful. It introduces another frightening question: will you ever have a perfect baby?

'*What are you making such a fuss about? Women are having miscarriages all the time.*'
But this is your miscarriage. It is a death which you need time and space to grieve over.

'*It doesn't matter so much to you because you already have a child.*'
This is another way of denying the way you feel and invalidating it.

'*At your age you can go on and have any number of babies.*'
Perhaps, but at the moment you are grieving over the loss of this particular one and prospective breeding abilities are irrelevant.

'*In your heart of hearts perhaps you didn't really want a baby now.*'
This is sheer cruelty. Many other women 'don't want a baby' at this stage of their lives, but still do not have miscarriages. You are being told that you killed your baby.

'*Take my advice. Try and forget about it. Keep busy and enjoy yourself.*'
You were not asking for advice. If you could do these things, you would.

'*It's just one of those things.*'
Doctors sometimes say this. Maybe they should say, 'I don't know' and 'I don't understand why'. Put like that, it becomes less personal and you are not likely to feel shrugged off and dismissed.

There is also the person who says, '*OK now?*', smiles nervously and hurries on to talk about other things. The message here is that she would rather not talk about it. You feel that you have committed a social solecism in having a miscarriage.

There is also the woman who cannot wait to tell you, '*When I had my miscarriage . . .*' The reality of your experience is rejected while she concentrates on the excitement of hers. It is true, though, that if you did not realise that she had ever had a miscarriage it can be comforting because you do not feel such a solitary failure.

If people never mention your miscarriage at all, that hurts too, and you feel deserted.

Some particular cheering information, long part of women's knowledge, is endorsed by doctors. If you suffer from nausea and vomiting in early pregnancy you are much less at risk of miscarriage than women who don't vomit. However, if you are pregnant and *not* vomiting, this does not mean that you are going to have a miscarriage!

You may be anxious about having intercourse in case it dislodges the developing embryo. The evidence that avoiding sex helps prevents miscarriage is rather shaky, though if not having intercourse helps you relax better, enjoy alternative kinds of lovemaking in the first few months of pregnancy.

There is no evidence that sex in pregnancy triggers miscarriage. But as you approach your 'due date' sexual activity may help open the cervix ready for dilatation. This does not necessarily involve penetration. Studies of nipple stimulation reveal that this is effective in ripening the cervix, and also reduces the rate of postpartum haemorrhage.[19]

Tiredness

Many women feel incredibly tired during the first weeks. They worry that they will be like this until they have the baby. Physical exhaustion is associated with the major adjustments the whole body is making in those first weeks. The baby is fully formed in miniature by three months and by this time, too, every cell in your body is involved in adapting to meet the challenge of pregnancy. No wonder you are tired!

Moreover, all this is happening when you may have told very few people about being pregnant, so no concessions are made when you feel under pressure at work, for example, or think you should finish something you have started by the time you are going to leave to have the baby. A woman who does not have a job outside the home, but who is busy with older children, may want to prove to herself that she is going to be able to handle the toddler and a baby, too. The result is that she drops into bed with relief and falls asleep as soon as she can. Sex is the last thing she wants.

A woman who feels confident about her sexuality and who normally enjoys it is more likely to take this in her stride. Studies also show that a woman having her first baby tends to be less interested in sex at the beginning of pregnancy, whereas women having second and subsequent babies often notice very little change in libido.

Some women actually enjoy sex more as soon as they know they are pregnant. It may sound odd, but they find it easier to give themselves to their feelings when they are pregnant because there is no longer the *risk* of getting pregnant. For them the whole business of contraception is associated with 'holding back', 'being careful', 'remembering' – to take the pill for example; with making sure that a condom hasn't slipped off as the man withdraws; with recording the menstrual cycle and having intercourse only when it is 'safe', or even gambling with getting the man out before he ejaculates. A woman who is constantly anxious about getting pregnant discovers that, once pregnant, she can forget all these things and relax and enjoy it.

Even so, this is more likely to happen after about 10 to 12 weeks. Sometimes it takes even longer to start to enjoy pregnancy. But once the period of nausea and vomiting, anxiety about possible miscarriage and extreme lassitude is over, many women say they enjoy sex more than ever before. The middle months of pregnancy are a time when they feel happy with their bodies and glow with a kind of pregnancy radiance.

This probably will not happen if you are under great pressure at work or if having a baby means that you are constantly worrying about money. In that case the fatigue felt in the first weeks tends to continue and you never get 'turned on' in mid-pregnancy. Nor is it likely to happen if you feel angry about being pregnant in the first place, or trapped by all kinds of obligations at work or in the family. Though some women actually enjoy 'angry' sex and repressed hostility seems to give lovemaking an extra zip, in pregnancy this kind of fighting lovemaking does not seem to work for most women and becomes merely painful. Your partner must change his ways of making love or you may want to avoid it altogether.

The Second Three Months

By the beginning of the fourth month tissues around and inside the vagina have 'ripened' and remain like this throughout pregnancy. William Masters and Virginia Johnson describe them, in *Human Sexual Response*, as engorged in a way similar to that during sexual arousal. They have become thicker and swollen, rather as a soft fruit ripens. Even the colour has changed from shades of pale pink and red to purple, violet and blue as a result of the increased blood supply. This means that a woman is in a permanent state of gentle sexual arousal. She also feels much more moist. Extra vaginal lubrication, which seeps through the convoluted walls of the vagina, may make her much more conscious of her vagina. Some women say they feel juicy and sweet.

The pressure on the genital organs from about the fourth month is so great for some women that they say they feel 'horny', like Jane, who admits, 'I can't wait for my husband to get home, poor man!' or Rosie, who says, 'I couldn't get through the day without masturbating, I feel so sexy. I thought I must be very peculiar until I talked to my sister-in-law about it. She had a baby last year and she said she felt just the same.'

A woman who is feeling super-charged like this can be aghast to discover that her partner does not want to have intercourse or is unable to get or maintain an erection. Many men are anxious that they can hurt the baby. This concern may have very good effects, because they become more considerate about lovemaking than before. But a man who is really frightened may refuse even to touch the woman. Some men have told me that they were terrified of breaking the bag of waters. Others believe that they can damage the baby. Others that if they let themselves go everything can get out of hand and labour may start immediately. It is almost as if they feel that by keeping themselves under restraint it will help make the pregnancy go well; as if their self-control will somehow 'guard' the pregnancy. These beliefs are remarkably similar to those held in traditional cultures, where taboos are enjoined on a father to ensure the well-being of a baby while it is still in the uterus.

Most couples probably find that they want to adapt lovemaking techniques as pregnancy advances. Any weight on the breasts feels extremely uncomfortable and the 'missionary position' is a very bad one unless a male partner is careful to take all his weight on his forearms. A side-lying position in which the woman has her back to the man as she nestles into his 'lap' is often comfortable for this reason. Some women enjoy being on all fours or kneeling with him behind.

Around 20 Weeks

Oxytocin levels rise during pregnancy. By 40 weeks a woman is usually feeling most self-confident and in the best health. She usually feels the baby's movements around 20 weeks and starts to have Braxton-Hicks contractions that tone the uterus. Elizabeth Davis describes it as a stage when many women experience increased libido. Alice, a mother of three, says: 'When it comes to sex, I also felt that I had more ability each time to communicate my knowledge of the baby to my partner. Our deep connection to one another during lovemaking began to include the baby, too, especially with the last. This was so wonderful – memories I will always treasure. I was with child and with the man I love, both at the same time. I felt completely fulfilled.'

Elizabeth Davis then goes on to say 'Take ample amounts of oxytocin, mix with high levels of estrogen, progesterone and vaginal engorgement, and no wonder many women in their second trimester find themselves sexually insatiable, surprising both themselves and their partners.'[20]

The Last Three Months

By about seven months, indigestion and heartburn may be a problem when you lie flat, so have your head and shoulders well raised with pillows. This means that you prefer making love in a sitting position, using a big floor cushion, a chair, or the side of the bed.

A woman's fantasies about her body – her body image – subtly affect her sexual feelings. The body is going through such vast changes during pregnancy that some women feel far bigger than they really are or believe that their partners must find them ugly, when, in fact, men often delight in pregnant women and find the physical changes exciting and beautiful. One woman described herself as like 'a hippopotamus wallowing in the mud' and said she felt completely sexless right through her pregnancy. Another said she felt like 'a goddess, queen of all dark growing things stirring deep in the earth'. She was in a state of erotic arousal until she went into labour, and kept that feeling through the birth.

Technocratic and authoritarian antenatal care can make it difficult for a woman to enjoy her body. It does so by conveying the message that the ordinary ways of knowing about and trusting our bodies are no longer valid and that we must defer to medical opinion and accept a medical view of what is happening to us. Women often go for an antenatal check-up with a sense of well-being, but leave feeling anxious, depressed or ill. The image of our bodies imposed on us can put an invisible brake on pleasure in sex.

This is particularly the case for a woman who is undergoing a series of special tests, including, for example, amniocentesis, serial ultrasound scans, oestriol tests and other investigations. She is more likely to have her whole pregnancy 'medicalised' when it has been difficult to start a baby in the first place or to hang on to a pregnancy. Then her relationship with her partner comes second to that with her obstetrician. It is as if the doctor and the pregnant patient form a new procreating couple and that the health and life of the baby depends on this. The baby's father may come to see himself as unnecessary and even as a danger to the fetus.

It is vital that a couple talk about this together and that expert professional care is not allowed to usurp or intrude on the special relationship of a couple who are becoming parents. Their responsibility for the baby continues long past the pregnancy and birth, and anything which adversely affects them can have long-term consequences for the child. Expectant parents need to be able to nurture each other in order to grow into being a mother and father capable, in their turn, of nurturing a baby.

A loving sexual relationship can contribute to the well-being of a pregnancy not only because the woman knows she is cherished and because the ordinary stresses of life are temporarily dissolved whenever she turns towards her lover, but because when she is sexually aroused oxytocin is released into her bloodstream. Dr Michel Odent calls it 'the happiness hormone'. Oxytocin is important in contributing to the good tone of the contracting uterus. Uterine sensitivity to oxytocin builds up in the last few weeks and this leads to the spontaneous start of labour.

When obstetricians induce labour they often use a synthetic form of oxytocin – Syntocinon. Or they may use prostaglandins in the form of a suppository inserted near the cervix. The highest natural concentration of prostaglandins in the human body is in semen.

If a baby is due to be born but labour has not been triggered spontaneously on the calculated date, passionate lovemaking can sometimes further soften the cervix and start contractions which initiate labour. Yet, faced with what they see as the threat of induction, many couples feel too intimidated to experiment with their own ways of inducing labour naturally.

Anxiety about induction also means that a woman may not feel like making love. It is as if she has already become the object of medical care, a uterus, a pelvis and birth canal to be acted on obstetrically, just at a time when lovemaking – and feeling a whole person – could contribute most to the natural flow of the birthing process. She may also draw back from intercourse because when the baby is deep in the pelvis it is often uncomfortable. It can feel as if the penis is perilously close to the baby's head. 'I felt that any violent, thrusting penile movements might be injurious to myself or my child', one woman says. 'I felt increasingly protective for the well-being of my baby, so much so that I felt the child's well-being far more important than whether my partner was satisfied or not after lovemaking.' In fact, the baby is well protected inside a membrane-walled bubble of water and the soft tissues of the cervix act as a cushion in front of its head, too.

Once the fetus has engaged in the pelvis, with its head fitting neatly into the bony cradle like an egg in an egg cup, it may feel as if the baby is about to drop out and there is no spare room. Even if you did not want it before, you may prefer a position in which your partner enters you from behind. When you lie, crouch or kneel with your back to him the uterus, which lies almost at a right angle to your vagina, is free from pressure and you can use your buttock muscles to grip the penis, so controlling the depth of penetration.

Elizabeth Davis writes that if lesbian mothers 'align with their partners hormonally – estrogen peaks and menses in synchrony – it makes possible an even deeper physical empathy in pregnancy that enables both parents to know the baby intimately, even though the nonpregnant partner has no biological link.'[21]

Encouraging Labour to Start

There is a special way of having intercourse if you want to start labour. It has not been subjected to controlled research, but experience shows that many women, either coincidentally or as a result, go into labour during the night following this kind of lovemaking. It will not always work, but gives you a chance of starting naturally.

Lie on your back, head and shoulders well supported by as many pillows as you like for comfort, your partner facing you and kneeling between your parted legs. Lift one leg so that your foot is over his shoulder. Then the other. Though this position is not comfortable, it allows the deepest penetration so that the tip of the penis can touch the cervix.

Though it is not necessary to have an orgasm, and being determined to achieve orgasm can make it more difficult to have one, if your partner knows how to touch you so that you become excited, too, and have an orgasm, it may start contractions which later settle into the rhythmic pattern of early labour. When he has ejaculated he should stay inside you for five minutes or so while you stay in the same position, with legs raised for 10 to 15 minutes, so that the cervix is bathed in semen.

Follow intercourse with manual and oral nipple stimulation. This is often effective even without intercourse. It is also helpful in labour if progress is very slow, or if contractions come to a stop, since stimuli received from the nipples trigger uterine contractions. About 20 minutes of nipple caressing, interspersed with other kinds of loving touch, seems right for most women.

Do not lie awake waiting for labour to start. Let yourself relax and drift off to sleep. Even if you do not start contracting, you have probably helped the cervix to ripen further.

One man described what happened in these words: 'Weak, irregular contractions started immediately after we had made love. When I sucked her nipples they got much stronger. I worked out that I could keep the contractions going by touching or licking her nipples about every ten minutes. Then she got up and walked around a little and I think that helped. But she was tired and wanted to get some sleep before starting, so I kept contractions going with nipple stimulation and she dozed between them. It was hard work, but I enjoyed it. I felt really useful because it was so obvious it was helping the labour.'

When we realise that pregnancy and birth are not primarily medical conditions, but part of a woman's psychosexual experience, we discover the relations between different aspects of our sexuality and gain new understanding, in touch with our bodies and our feelings.

4

ACTIVE BIRTH-GIVING

Hormones

Hormones are chemical messengers in the bloodstream and play an important part in sexual arousal and the physical changes that go with it, and also in birth. Like the nervous system, and in partnership with it, they keep the whole organism developing and functioning as an entity, right through our lives. They link up different parts of our bodies, co-ordinating them into a whole, making us individuals – not just a set of disconnected organs. Hormones span the invisible space between mind and body.

They are secreted by the endocrine glands which keep our bodies working normally. The egg follicle of the ovary and the placenta, the tree of life for a developing fetus, are temporary endocrine glands, while the pituitary gland, at the base of the brain, is a permanent gland.

Some hormones, for example those secreted by the thyroid gland in the neck, affect every cell in our bodies. Others serve specific organs. Ovaries secrete oestrogen which has a specific action on our genitals and breasts, and also maintains the health of skin, mucus membranes and other body tissues.

Our ovaries manufacture progesterone as well as oestrogen. These are both steroids – hormones derived from cholesterol. Every steroid can be changed into another by the action of enzymes, which are soluble proteins produced by living cells to act as catalysts.

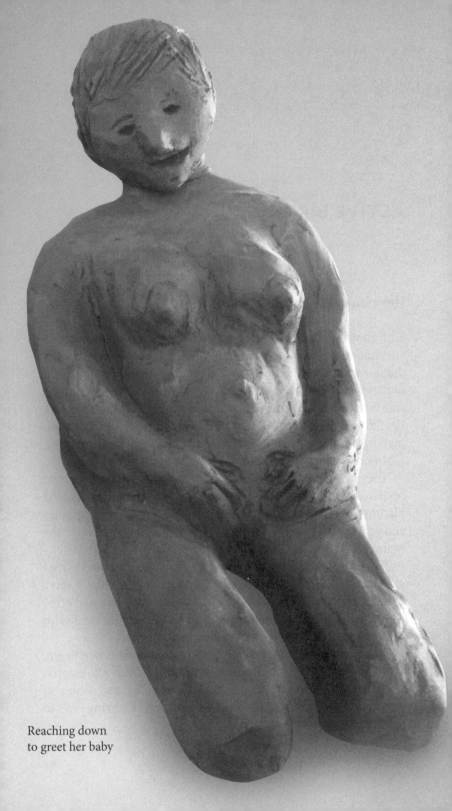

Reaching down
to greet her baby

Oestrogen plays an important role in our bodies through all the changes of puberty, menstruation and pregnancy. It is produced every month by the ripening egg follicle, and levels change at various times in the cycle.

Progesterone is also secreted in a monthly rhythm. It is vital to ovulation, the rebuilding of the lining of the uterus once a period is over, and to enrich the wall of the uterus so that it provides a nourishing 'broth' for a fertilised ovum to feed on.

Oestrogen reaches its peak just before ovulation. After a period is over the oestrogen level rises again. It stimulates the cervix to secrete mucus which is at first thick, sticky and opaque, but which gradually changes and gets thin, slippery, clear and stretchy, like raw egg white. Once mucus is like this it enables sperm to swim easily through up into the cervix, and from there into the uterus and fallopian tubes.

After ovulation the level of oestrogen drops steeply. Progesterone thickens the mucus again to form a plug in the cervix until the next period begins. With menstruation levels of both oestrogen and progesterone drop. Without hormonal support, the surface of the uterine lining disintegrates and is discharged with the menstrual period.

Medical books usually take a 28-day cycle as the norm. But a woman can be perfectly healthy and have a cycle which is of a different pattern. If you are under stress, or not having good nutrition, your cycle may change dramatically. When you come off the contraceptive pill it can be about a year, sometimes even longer, before the cycle develops a regular pattern again.

Changes in the Vaginal Mucus

Natural secretions keep the vagina moist and clean and you can get to know where you are in your menstrual cycle by knowing the state of the mucus. In the first days after a period there may be very little mucus and the vagina feels dry. That usually lasts five to seven days. Then a thick, non-stretchy mucus starts to flow from the cervix.

As oestrogen rises the mucus changes and becomes watery and stretchy. Your vagina feels slippery and wet. There may be glistening mucus on your pants. Taking some between your thumb and forefinger, it can stretch up to four inches. Occasionally it is pink because of the presence of blood. This is highly fertile mucus. Ovulation occurs when there are copious quantities of this type of mucus.

The mucus stays thick and sticky for a day or two. This is followed by a run of dry days until the next period begins. Some women notice a thickening of mucus just before a period comes. But you can have cycles in which no ovum ripens, or you may ovulate more than once in a cycle. The general pattern, however, is that an ovum becomes ripe at three- to six-week intervals.

Birth and the Endocrine System

Birth should not be summed up in terms of sheer pain, as a demonstration of self-control, or a physiological performance in which a woman puts on an exhibition of athletic breathing skills. In an environment where she knows that she is free to be spontaneous, supported by relationships which enable her to release and trust her body, hormones flow in her bloodstream with the same energy as in ecstatic lovemaking. Birth and sex mingle to become one in the thrilling, sweet, intense and overwhelming experience of creation. It can be mind-blowing and orgasmic.

In the course of her sexual response cycle when she is making love a woman passes through an *excitement phase* that may last hours or a matter of minutes. Her breasts enlarge, the tissues over the centre of her abdomen flush, and this may spread over the breasts as well. Her blood pressure and heart rate increase. Masters and Johnson analysed this response in detail back in the 1960s.[22] The clitoris swells, both in length and diameter. The walls of the vagina are moistened and lubricated by fluid that flows from enlarged blood vessels, passing through the connective tissue and epithelium of the vaginal wall. As a result the uterus tips forward.[23]

A similar excitement phase occurs when a woman wants to push during labour. It is an intricately co-ordinated interplay of sensations and responses, one that is destroyed if she feels under threat – whether that is because she is being helped in an inappropriate and bossy way, focused on critically, or simply told what to do and expected to obey.

It is not a matter of the sudden, explosive orgasm which is typical for a man, but much more subtle than that. Hormonal waves in the bloodstream stimulate birth and sexual experience generally. They do not trigger instant orgasms.

In the medical management of birth giving 'help' often means that the mother has unnecessary interference and is forced to conform to superimposed instructions and to what amounts to a threat. This stimulates the production of adrenaline and a reaction of 'fight or flight'.

It is vital to avoid disturbing a woman in childbirth. Michel Odent has pointed out that this is the most important element in giving support.[24] Though managing birth is often disguised as helping, it is an expression of the attendant's own anxiety, and can have disastrous consequences. Spontaneous birth does not result from neocortical activity, but from *instinct*. It is the same with all mammals:

'Asking the mother questions, constant verbal coaching, side conversations in the room, clicking cameras – there are so many ways to draw the mother from her ancient brain trance (necessary for a smooth expulsion of the baby) into the present-time world.'[25]

Mavis Kirkham believes that the second stage of labour is a bad time for discussion. The mental work does not help a woman in strong labour: 'In active labour without an epidural, discussion of a woman's needs and choices is difficult and can be counterproductive.'[26]

The Climax of Birth

To experience the sexuality of birth you need to 'run wild'. It is not enough to relax. Only when we surrender neocortical domination and let our bodies work freely can we give birth as other mammals do, without self-consciousness and inhibition.

'Since I had heard that staying loose in the mouth would keep the cervix loose during each intense sensation that came, I grabbed my husband . . . and kissed him. We didn't just kiss, our mouths were wide and smooching. The more intense the feelings, the more intense the kissing. It was wonderful. Labour lasted four hours, and with three pushes, Giacomo was out.'

'He was reclining next to me, and at the start of a heavy contraction, I found his mouth. We French kissed. Whew! Here comes another! We kissed again, from the start to the finish of the contraction.'[27]

In spontaneous vaginal birth as the baby slides out the mother's levels of adrenaline and noradrenaline are high. They give her the energy to push. Immediately after, levels plummet if she is feeling safe, private and undisturbed, and is able to reach out and focus on her baby.[28] But if she is actively managed in the third stage and feels the need to be vigilant, these fight or flight hormones remain high, and may even rise further. Moreover, if the baby is not in skin-to-skin contact with her and is taken to be processed by caregivers the flow of oxytocin is reduced.

The baby in her arms seeks her breast and nuzzles it to initiate suckling. This stimulates the limbic system in her brain, which activates her parasympathetic nervous system and creates feelings 'of calm and connection'. Sarah Buckley notes that 'These postnatal peaks of oxytocin also activate the "maternal circuit" in the new mother's brain, which is responsible for switching on instinctive mothering behaviour in all mammals.'[29] Her uterus contracts in response to these high levels of oxytocin, so there is less chance of heavy bleeding. If the mother and baby are separated bonding can be affected for as long as a year or more.

The same oxytocin-induced feelings of 'calm' and 'connection' are experienced after orgasm, and there are parallels in the feelings of euphoria after giving birth and the sense of well-being after sex.

In this way the intense sensuality and sexuality of birth stimulate babies to seek their mothers and empower women to love their babies.

Going Wild

To be wild, to roar like a lion, to scale mountains, and to revel in the birth passion, we need to feel we are in control of the place of birth, the people who support us, and anything that is done to us.

Research into self-control reveals that women often seek to control themselves and escape from their bodies, even want to hide them from care-givers, due to feelings of inadequacy, disappointment, frustration, and dissatisfaction with themselves and their bodies.[30] They do not want to 'lose control' and go wild. It is an attempt at de-sexing birth – and often proves successful. Only when a woman feels safe and private can she dare to surrender control completely.

Wanting to have control in childbirth is quite different from *self-control*. When we seek control over the environment in which we give birth it should be about choosing the people who attend us and what is done to us. Whereas for some women self-control – not yelling, guarding their behaviour, being completely rational and putting on a superb performance, is the priority, it de-sexes birth and makes it impossible to respond spontaneously to intense sensations, and be in touch with their instincts and the natural rush of hormones sweeping in the bloodstream in wave after wave of passion.

Birth is a psychosexual act in which a woman needs to be free to move her pelvis in response to waves of desire stimulated by a rush of hormones in her bloodstream. This is not merely a matter of being upright rather than supine.

Positions for delivery in traditional cultures were first recorded by Dr George Engelmann and a medical student, Robert Felkin, who described them in North American native cultures and African tribes in the nineteenth century. But information about how women *move* in labour has been patchy. Yet all over the world pelvic mobility and ways of encouraging this by providing physical support, and free movements that constitute, in effect, a birth dance, are practised, in stark contrast to the immobility usually imposed on women in a technocratic birth culture, where they are expected to lie on a bed or delivery table.

Before the delivery table was invented women were often upright or semi-upright as they moved. They stood, squatted, leant half-squatting, grasped stakes set in the ground or the central house pole, or held on to a rope or a long strip of cloth suspended from a beam, and knotted at the lower end. Often another woman, or sometimes the father of the baby, held the mother from behind and moved with her. A further variation was when she stood with a woman at either side, arms around her, who moved in synchrony with her.

A combination of having a bar or pole to grasp and walking around between contractions was common. In Montana the Flathead woman grasped a horizontal bar fixed between two upright posts so she could rock her pelvis, and gave birth leaning against another woman on a skin spread with soft bison wool. In Central Africa the Banyoro alternatively grasped a stick driven into the ground and walked in a circle round it. Japanese women traditionally adopted many different positions for the second stage. The mother held on to a rope hanging from the ceiling, and moved between half-sitting and standing. She might kneel leaning against a pile of straw bundles and a quilt, sit leaning back with the midwife or her husband holding her pelvis from behind, crouch forward over a bag of rice, or kneel with her back supported by futons. There are myths that one Empress gave birth to twins while leaning against a mortar, and that another delivered her son while holding on to a branch of the pagoda tree at a shrine.[31]

When a woman laboured out of doors in the New Guinea forest or the African bush she walked around and grasped the

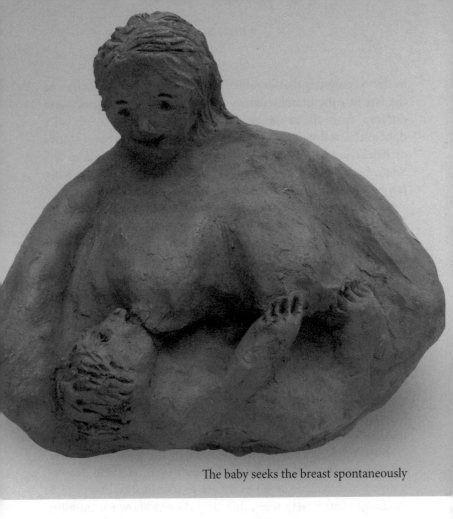

The baby seeks the breast spontaneously

trunk or branch of a tree as each contraction came.

Among some native North Americans it was the practice to erect a palisade of branches with stakes pushed into the ground at measured intervals, forming a path into an inner sanctum. The woman walked from stake to stake as her labour progressed. It provided visible evidence of the advance of her labour, and when she entered the second stage at last she reached the inner space where she could give birth.

A Hopi woman squatted or knelt on a sheepskin in the corner of the birth room, and walked around between contractions. Bedouin Arab girls learned pelvic movements for sex and birth in the ceremonies that heralded adulthood. This is the origin of the North African belly dance. It is slow and languorous, quite different from the rapid gyrations and jerks of night-club belly dancing. Kneeling was often made easier by using birth stones or bricks, and the woman was free to move her pelvis as she knelt. In Egypt women knelt on two birth stones. In the King James Bible this was interpreted as 'stools': 'And the King of Egypt spoke to the Hebrew midwives . . . And he said, When ye do the office of a midwife to the Hebrew women and see them upon the stools . . .' It was a loose rendering of an Egyptian word that meant 'a pair of stones'. Kneeling on them, a woman rocked back and forth.

An alternative was to sit between the thighs of another woman. Rachel says of the labour of her maid servant, Bilha, 'She shall bear upon my knees that I may also have children by her.'

American archaeologists discovered some birth bricks from ancient Egypt in 2002 in a palace that was 3700 years old. They excavated an elaborately decorated and colourful birth brick that shows a mother with her newborn, attended on either side by helping women and by Hathor, the Cow Goddess of birth and motherhood.[32]

Birth bricks are still used by women in India. Nowadays they are ordinary builder's bricks, which they even take into hospital with them. Unaccustomed as we are to hammocks, except to lie in the garden, it may seem that they do not allow for mobility. But in South America babies are conceived, cradled and born in hammocks. They are cheap, familiar, flexible, washable, biodegradable, and can be adapted to different activities. In the Amazon, tribal women give birth in a closely woven cotton hammock into which a large hole has been cut and the baby drops through it onto warm, soft ashes or into a water-filled canoe. In Mexico and Guatemala a woman gives birth in her old hammock, with a new hammock hanging above it on which she pulls during contractions. After the birth the old hammock is discarded and she and the baby move into the new one.

In Europe birth stools are not mentioned until the second century AD, when they are referred to in the very first obstetric textbook. Throughout North Africa and Europe the mother sat on a birth stool and women helpers offered their own bodies to support the mother from behind. Only later were backs constructed for these stools. At first they were sloped so that the woman could move her pelvis. But already by the sixteenth century in Germany they had turned into birth chairs, and it was the midwife who sat on the stool in front of the woman. The more elaborate birth chairs became, the more difficult it was for the woman to move. She was more or less upright, but fixed in one position. In the fourteenth century Haggadah of Sarajevo miniature paintings show the birth of Rebecca's twins with the mother sitting on a birth stool and the midwife kneeling at her feet. In the sixteenth century German illustrations depict women sitting on elaborate birth chairs with a midwife either sitting on a stool or kneeling at their feet, always with other women attending. In the nineteenth century the Prussian consul in Jerusalem wrote that peasant women gave birth on stones, but wealthier women used birth chairs.

Today women are rediscovering the advantages of pelvic movement during labour and rather than using special equipment for support, hold on to furniture, a partner, or if they give birth at home, even a tree in the garden. In hospital a hammock or cloth sling attached to a strong hook in the ceiling enables a woman to use gravity to help her bear down and to move the lower part of her body freely. The hammock needs to be fixed so that it can be raised or lowered, depending on how she wishes to use it.[33]

As European and American obstetrics spread to South America, Africa and beyond in the twentieth century medicalised birth was superimposed on traditional cultures, and caregivers went to great lengths to ensure that women obeyed instructions and adapted to the 'modern' 'scientific' way. With the invention of the delivery table they were prevented from moving and fixed to a metal slab. The positions imposed upon them were designed to make the uterus and vulva easily accessible for the obstetrician to employ manoeuvres of various kinds – each of which was labelled in the textbooks with the name of the obstetrician who originally devised it.

An English medical student who did an elective in Algeria described an event in the hospital delivery room:

It's her eighth delivery, and her first in hospital. This time, she says, she felt 'tired'. She's been in labour all night. Her cervix is fully open and the baby's head is where it should be, ready to come down. But something's wrong. Her contractions are short and weak. She doesn't seem to have her heart in the whole business. Djamila [the midwife] wags her finger and threatens the woman in French, which she doesn't understand: 'If you're not careful, Dr Kostov will come and give you a big spanking.' She gets up on the bed and kneels beside the woman, pressing down on her belly with both hands, arms stiff and straight, trying to push the baby out. To no avail. We go out onto the landing to rest.

We come back to find the woman squatting on the floor, holding herself upright by the bed post. Fatma the Kabyl cleaner screams. Djamila spits Arab war-cries. They shoo the woman back on to the bed. Djamila won't hear of delivering her on the floor. She's scandalised. She's never seen it done, but she knows there must be a good reason against it. Women deliver on their backs, all else is primitive.

On the bed the woman looks solemnly at Djamila. Then she flicks her thumb nail against her front teeth at her. Djamila's wounded, and she falls onto the chair in the corner. She'll have nothing more to do with the woman, who's telling Fatma that she won't go anywhere else but the floor. She always squatted before, and that's what she's going to do now. If they won't let her, she's going to sleep. She stretches out her legs, throws down her robe and closes her eyes.[34]

During field work in Moscow in the 1970s I witnessed how, after the ritual complete shave and enema, the woman was put on a narrow, hard, high bed to 'get on with it'. She lay alone, biting her lips, moaning quietly, or writhing in silent agony. When it was judged time for the baby to be born she was wheeled to the delivery room and had to climb on a table, lie flat on her back, push as hard as she could, and there was a hurried, violent delivery conducted by an obstetrician.

This is how the second stage is managed in hospitals all over the world where midwifery is not strong, practice is not evidence-based, and the primary concern of caregivers is to tether the mother in a position convenient for obstetric manoeuvres so that she cannot possibly move away.

Obstetric equipment firms compete energetically to market ever more elaborate delivery tables and birth chairs. At any international obstetric or birth conference they can be seen crowding the exhibition hall. I usually kick off my shoes and try them all. There is a state-of-the-art Italian birth chair constructed of stainless steel and black rubber, advertised as providing 'the most favourable position for physiological deliveries'. This turns out to be the woman reclining on her back, legs raised in lithotomy stirrups, wrists and ankles cuffed, and shoulders restrained to prevent her from moving her head. She looks as if she is in the grip of a giant tarantula. Malvestio, the manufacturing company, promotes it this way: 'Because of its mobility this equipment allows the obstetrician to effectively and rationally intervene on the expectant mother' and with pressure on a button that produces 'a single fast clutch-operated movement' the chair will transform into a table on which a Caesarean section can be performed. The equipment can be rapidly adjusted – the woman remains immobilised. But protest against being tethered in such a way is building up across the world.

The Right to Move

Being free to move is important to women. They don't want to be fettered or stuck in a position from which they cannot escape. They refuse to be placed like a lab specimen, legs splayed under a bright light.

When in 1982 the Senior Lecturer in Obstetrics at London's prestigious Royal Free Hospital, Yehudi Gordon, was ordered by the Professor not to allow women to sit up, kneel, squat, or adopt other upright or semi-upright positions to give birth, women rallied to defend him. It was rather like being told that the missionary position was the only one permitted for sex.[35]

A group of women in the birth movement got together to organise a public demonstration outside the hospital. The night before, I had a call from the Director of Crowd Control at Scotland Yard, who told me that we could not meet outside the hospital because there was no space for the masses who were going to turn up. So I arranged a march from the hospital to Parliament Hill Fields with the police escorting us, some on foot and others mounted.

Five thousand people joined us – pregnant women, mothers and babies, their partners, midwives, medical students and other professionals. They stepped off coaches that came from all parts of the country. There were teenagers and white-haired women, many with babies in slings against their bodies, or in strollers or prams.

Afterwards the Professor of Obstetrics resigned. He explained that it was nothing to do with the demonstration, and went off to specialise in *in vitro* fertilisation.

Since then women have been able to move when and how they wish and give birth in upright positions in that hospital. It has had a knock-on effect in other hospitals, too, and it is now generally accepted in the UK that women do not have to give birth lying flat on their backs or with legs splayed in lithotomy stirrups.

5

ACTIVE MANAGEMENT

'Active management' was first introduced in Dublin by O'Driscoll in the 1960s. Obstetric efficiency experts, obeying strict protocols, were to get women's bodies running like well oiled machines and babies to emerge safely as if from a production line, without wasting doctors' time, and free of any female emotions that might complicate the process. He offered 'military efficiency with a human face'.[36] With active management a woman is recorded as in labour from the moment she is examined and admitted to hospital. What she says she is feeling is irrelevant. The medical team must keep control over labour and each birth is normal only in retrospect.

The underlying assumption of active management is that every phase of birth, every contraction, the dilatation of the cervix, and the expulsion of the fetus and placenta, should conform to a time-limited linear pattern. That, in turn, depends on strict recording of each element of labour on a chart, followed by a diagnosis of normality or abnormality. For the diagnosis of normality dilatation should be at least one centimetre per hour.

It was Emanuel Friedmann, a mathematician who made a career switch to medicine, who came up with that idea. His wife was having a baby in the hospital where he worked as a junior obstetrician. Fathers were not allowed to be present at births, so he was at a loose end while she was in labour, and to control his anxiety he went round the wards performing an anal examination on women every half-hour to check that the cervix was dilating and recording the time it took. He came up with a graph.

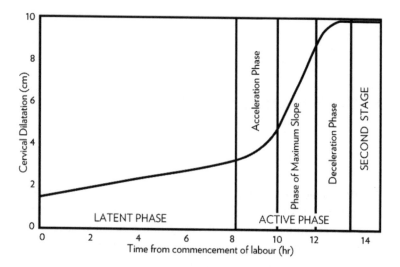

If the measurement did not sit on the statistical curve that represented the mean it was an 'abnormal' labour, whatever the outcome. Examinations performed like that frequently have the effect of stimulating painful contractions and artificially forcing dilatation. The model he produced was based on labours in which a woman was constantly poked about.

Clock-Dominated Birth

In agricultural societies work is linked to the seasons. As winter gives way to spring, spring to summer, then autumn and winter again, workers use different skills, and tasks change their patterns of interaction.

With the industrial revolution linear, or clock, time replaced this. In Belgium, where the railway was invented, its schedules across Europe were the basis for this concept of time. Now births are regulated by the clock. Any labour that does not fit strict guidelines is abnormal. Consequently women worry when they feel 'practice' contractions of the uterus in the second half of pregnancy and if they go past the 'due date'. Their expectations and fears may alert them to ask for labour to be induced, and as more and more labours take place within this narrow band of time, a clock-time view of pregnancy is reinforced.[37]

Midwives who resist the technology of surveillance may seek to protect women from it and avoid handing them over to obstetricians.[38] They then intervene themselves in a less drastic way – dosing women with castor oil, giving them an enema, sweeping the membranes, or advising sexual activity to get labour started, for instance.

Labour, too, is circumscribed by strict time limits. *Myles' Midwifery*, the standard textbook, states that the active phase 'proceeds at a rate of 1 to 1.5 cm per hour'.[39]

In Dublin every pregnant woman was presented with a partogram 'the focus of antenatal preparation for labour' when admitted to hospital so that they knew why they were being monitored minutely and their position on the graph.[40] As a consequence women in labour asked midwives and doctors, 'How long have I got?'[41] Christine McCourt concludes that time in childbirth 'is physiological, psychological and social in the way that it is experienced and framed. The ways in which time . . . is conceptualised and managed enact social and cultural relationships of power and . . . institutionalise them.'[42]

The Active Management Epidemic

Active management spread like wild fire around the world wherever Western-style medicalised childbirth had been introduced, but lacked the one-to-one care which was a vital element in the Dublin method. It continues to be the basis of technocratic childbirth. The de-sexing of childbirth is complete.

In Dublin the rule was one-to-one nursing, strict time-keeping, a progress chart to which labour must conform, and firm discipline. Any woman who lost control and made a noise or behaved emotionally was accused of being selfish. Antenatal classes were introduced as a means of training women to conform to this system.

As one obstetrician put it in a book addressed to mothers, 'You will learn to adapt to the difficulties and to accept the changes that occur. You will learn to co-operate with your professional advisors'.[43] It was completely different from Dick-Read's approach to antenatal education which came later, and aimed for birth free from fear, helping women work with their bodies.

Active management entails induction if a woman is more than a week or so past the due date, electronic monitoring of the fetal heart with an electrode stuck through her vagina into the baby's scalp, and the control of uterine activity by a hormone intravenous drip so that labour is not allowed to exceed 12 hours, 10 hours, eight hours, or whatever the obstetrician has decided is the correct norm for dilatation and expulsion. If the baby is not born within the time limit set, delivery is achieved by forceps or Caesarean section.

O'Driscoll aimed to cut the Caesarean rate, but instead active management pushed it higher, because artificial stimulation of the uterus made contractions more painful, women had more drugs for pain relief, and epidural rates went up.

Epidural anaesthesia offered what is, for some women, painless childbirth, though the mother's blood pressure may drop suddenly and she may develop a fever, both of which can make her feel ill. Once she has an indwelling catheter in her spine, a woman can have all sensation removed from her waist down, though labour may be long and drawn out and the baby might get stuck with its head unable to rotate. If she chooses, and her anaesthetist times it correctly, some sensation can be allowed to return for the expulsive stage of labour so that she has more chance of being able to push her baby out. Even so, the need for forceps delivery, though it may be only a simple 'lift out', or vacuum extraction using strong suction, is increased with an epidural. A study by I J Hoult, A H MacLennan and L E Carrie 'Lumbar epidural analgesia in labour', revealed that women are five times more likely to have an operative delivery after this form of anaesthesia.[44] It puts extra stress on the perineum, and with the tissues around and inside her vagina ripped or sliced open she must be sutured, which may lead to sexual problems and subsequent incontinence.

As techniques have developed, epidural anaesthesia has been given with more discretion, so that, for example, a woman may be able to retain feeling in her legs, and with more experience with epidurals, among some obstetricians forceps rates have gone down. With others rates continue to rise.

An epidural is the most efficient method of removing pain with minimal effects on the fetus. The mother can read a magazine or do crossword puzzles through contractions and deliver while watching the birth as if on a television screen. She is calm, cool, collected – a fully 'co-operative patient'. And that is how epidural anaesthesia is promoted to obstetricians: it 'preserves the morale and co-operation of the mother', though they are warned that 'facilities for supportive measures to maintain vital functions such as maintenance of the airway, oxygenation with or without assisted ventilation, maintenance of blood pressure, etc, are essential', and such side effects as a sudden drop in blood pressure, 'tremor, tachycardia (a speeded up heart rate), bradycardia (a slowed down heart rate), malaise, vomiting and, rarely, convulsions or coma' may result.[45] But there is another price to pay, too. When physical sensation is obliterated birth is drained of all sexual feeling.

The vogue for induction, with artificial rupture of the membranes and an intravenous oxytocin drip, reached a peak in the early 1970s when, in many hospitals, nearly half of all births were kick-started in this way. It was not the only method of induction. Japanese obstetricians often prescribed electronic stimulation in the form of a small device pushed into the vagina that whirred rather like a miniature vacuum cleaner. These methods have largely been replaced by the use of prostaglandin suppositories inserted so that they press against the cervix.

Continuous electronic fetal monitoring also contributes to the de-sexing of childbirth. The equipment is fixed to the woman's body, both outside and inside. She is tethered by catheters and electric wires to equipment standing around the bed. She cannot move freely or even shift position without risking interfering with the printout of the monitor or detaching an electrode or indwelling catheter. It is almost as if it is the monitor which is having the baby, and all eyes are fixed on it.

The book that first raised important questions about all interventions and pointed the way to research into the risks and benefits of active management was *A Guide to Effective Care in Pregnancy and Childbirth.*[46] The authors exposed the patriarchal power of active management and the lack of research evidence for many routine practices.

The principle of 'first do no harm' is easily overlooked as researchers investigating new technologies test the efficacy of an intervention. 'The authoritative nature of the technocratic approach to birth has led to an over emphasis on the tools and techniques of this method, often without good evidence. Risk management has become a guiding force . . .' They point out that a randomised controlled trial, the best method of determining whether an intervention is effective on a population basis, is not necessarily the best way of discovering potential harm. 'Once an intervention has been introduced, it would seem that, while it would one day be replaced by a "better" intervention, it is rare that a decision is made that non-intervention is, after all, preferable.'[47]

The Birth Experience

It is against the background of the progressive depersonalisation of care, the takeover by machines and a cultural de-sexing of birth, that more and more women seek today to experience childbirth as a life-enhancing personal experience in which they can get in touch with their own feelings and give glad expression to the energy sweeping through their bodies. They are no longer so concerned about being 'in control' or proving that they have learned their exercises well. They are reclaiming the sexuality of childbirth.

This is highly disconcerting for those doctors who see their main service to patients as having 'a live mother and live baby', reducing the pain of labour, and cutting the time it takes. They are bewildered by women who want to move, to rock or crawl or dance, to be held in a lover's arms and embraced and kissed during labour, be stroked and massaged, and make whatever noises come naturally, whether it is to groan or sing, moan, or cry out. They feel rejected, as if the woman's complete involvement with what is happening implies hostility when they most want to help and to offer the patient their professional expertise.

In hospitals today there is more flexibility than even five years ago about what a woman can do during the first stage of labour, and when the cervix is dilating midwives often encourage her to walk around and get in any positions in which she is comfortable. In practice it is impossible to do this if she has continuous electronic fetal monitoring, but it is increasingly recognised that there is a physiological advantage – the uterus contracts better, the woman experiences less pain and the oxygen supply to the fetus is improved – when she can move freely. Traditional midwives working in cultures where technology has not taken over childbirth have always recognised this and encouraged and often shared in the uninhibited movement. As a Mexican midwife explained to me, 'We swing along'.[48]

Approaches to the Second Stage

The second stage of labour, however, when the baby is being pushed down the birth canal, is still treated as a time when a woman is supposed to battle with her body to get the baby born and to obey instructions she is given by her attendants. It is when we look at the second stage of labour that we realise just how far women in Western society have been turned into objects on which doctors act, and how much midwives have been trained in the medical model. For it is then that the basic lack of confidence in our bodies is expressed most clearly. The second stage is often turned into an athletic contest in which the woman struggles to push the baby down through the barriers of flesh, spurred on by everyone present. They form a cheerleading team urging her to greater effort, more sustained and deeper breaths, more energetic straining.

This not only makes her feel that she is falling short of a standard impossible to attain, but imposes unnecessary stress on the second stage which can adversely affect the baby. When a woman is exhausted with straining, bursts blood vessels in her face and eyes and tries to hold her breath for as long as possible, there is a risk that the cardiovascular disturbance created in her body will affect the baby's heart rate, its oxygen supply and acid base balance, according to a study done by Roberto Caldeyro-Barcia.[49] When she holds her breath and strains for a long time her blood pressure drops. This reduces the oxygen available to the baby. Then, when she can push no longer, she gasps for air and her blood pressure suddenly shoots up above normal. Yet long before this stage is reached the flow of oxygenated blood to the fetus may already be reduced. What often happens then is that dips in the fetal heart rate which persist after the end of the contraction are the signal for staff to urge her to push harder and hold her breath longer. This has the effect of cutting down the baby's oxygen supply still further.

Childbirth education classes must bear a good deal of responsibility for the strenuous pushing and prolonged breath-holding imposed on women in labour, who are being trained to do something which is quite unnatural. They have also often been taught how to strengthen and pull in their abdominal muscles. A woman who is tightening her abdominal muscles also pulls in her pelvic floor, resisting the descent of the baby's head and causing herself unnecessary pain. For the pelvic floor muscles are completely released only when the lower abdomen is allowed to bulge out, the very opposite of the muscular sucking-in movement still taught in some antenatal classes.

Other mammals do not behave like this. They do not get into the extraordinary positions which are often required of women in labour, lying flat on their backs with their legs up in the air in lithotomy stirrups, for example. They do not go in for all the huffing and puffing and breath-holding which women are taught to do. A cat or dog pushes its young out with short, rapid breaths and an open mouth. They also tend to choose a semi-upright position with the pelvis tilted and move around and shift position frequently during the expulsive stage.

When a woman does what comes naturally she breathes in very much the same way as other mammals giving birth. It is a breathing pattern which corresponds almost exactly to that of sexual excitement and orgasm. And she does this quite spontaneously. Masters and Johnson point out that during orgasm breathing is at least three times faster than the normal rate.[50] As a woman reaches the peak of orgasm her breath is involuntarily held and she gasps, groans, sighs or cries out. When it fades away her breathing gets slower again. If she is experiencing a multiple orgasm (waves of desire and fulfilment, with intervals between each), her breathing accelerates as each fresh wave rises in crescendo and then, as it peaks, she holds her breath for a few seconds – and may do this between one and five times at the height of orgasm. She then continues breathing quickly again and it gets slower as the orgasm wave passes.

This is how she breathes when she feels free to be spontaneous in the expulsive phase of labour. If she has never been to antenatal classes and is not told at the time how she should breathe or what she should do, she breathes quickly, holds her breath only for a few seconds, breathes out, continues to breathe quickly, holds her breath again for a few more seconds, and so on until the contraction starts to fade. And just like a woman having an orgasm, she wants to hold her breath like this between one and five times at the height of the contraction.

All this is quite different from the pattern usually imposed on women by instructions and the kind of encouragement they are given: 'Push! Push! Don't waste your contraction! . . . Take a deep breath, hold it. Now come on, you can do better than that! Don't let your breath go! Take another one! Hold it for as long as you can! . . . Breathe in, block, fix your ribs and diaphragm and push, 1-2-3-4-5-6-7-8-9-10.' The idea behind this is that she should be pushing right through a contraction, using every second of it, and putting her utmost strength into it.

It is the exact opposite of the female orgasm. What has happened is that a *male* model of physiological activity is being imposed on women in childbirth. The pattern of male orgasm – stiffen, hold, force through, shoot! – is distorting her own spontaneous psychosexual behaviour. Instead of the wave-like rhythms of female orgasm, bearing down is treated like one long ejaculation. A woman is supposed to carry on as long as she possibly can, and then sink back, exhausted. Any sexual feelings are completely eradicated. She is instructed to 'push into your bottom', or even 'Get angry with your baby!'

When she is pushing because it is insisted she does so, or because she believes it is the only way to get the baby out, stress is put on her perineum as the ball of the baby's head is propelled down through tissues which have not yet fanned out. And she is under great psychological stress as she struggles to expel the fetus as if trying to force out a large, hard, constipated motion.

6

EPISIOTOMY

The Active Management of Labour[51] is an attack on sexuality, with interventions that can have grave psycho-physical consequences. Episiotomy is a prime example of this: 'Just a little episiotomy', 'Better to have a nice straight cut than a nasty jagged tear', or as my midwife ordered me during my first home birth, in France, 'Push or I'll cut you.' So I pushed though I didn't want to – and tore.

The incision of a woman's perineum to enlarge the vagina is the most commonly performed obstetric operation in the West. An episiotomy is often done as part of the routine management of labour. Until recently some hospitals had close on 100 per cent rates. It is the only surgical intervention that takes place on the body of a healthy woman without her consent, and sometimes without informing her, as part of the active management of the second stage.

At the beginning of the 1970s I studied the effects of episiotomy and examined the responses to nearly 2,000 questionnaires completed by women who had attended National Childbirth Trust classes who gave birth over a period of one year.[52] It was preceded by a computer search of the medical literature, which revealed that even then the claims that episiotomy prevents prolapse, heals more easily than a tear, protects the baby's head from injury, and avoids other lacerations, were unsubstantiated. When I analysed the results of my survey – the first ever investigation made within the NCT – I discovered that a tear was almost always better for the mother than an episiotomy. At the end of the first week after birth, for example, women with natural lacerations had less pain than those with episiotomies. Twenty-three per cent of the episiotomy group had pain with intercourse lasting longer than three months, compared with 14 per cent of those with lacerations, and only two per cent of those with intact perineums. Cutting an incompletely dilated perineum increased blood loss and ripped tissue. Nearly half the episiotomies were done within 30 minutes of the beginning of the second stage of labour, before the perineum had time to fan out.

This was followed by a randomised controlled trial conducted by Jenny Sleep, a Reading midwife. She showed that a policy of performing episiotomies to prevent tears means unnecessary pain, stitches and infection. As soon as she started her research project – even before the results were published – midwives in her hospital began thinking about why they were so quick to cut, and the episiotomy rate went down dramatically.[53]

Over the next few years randomised controlled trials of episiotomy were conducted in the USA, the UK and some other Western countries.

At the West London Hospital in Hammersmith an obstetrician, Michael House, undertook research on episiotomies. He found that there was little to choose between an episiotomy and a second-degree tear. (Most tears are first-degree, nicks in the skin, whereas second-degree tears go into muscle.) He also discovered that women are much more likely to lose a large amount of blood when they have had an episiotomy. Again, there was an immediate drop of 30 per cent in the overall rate.[54]

Obstetricians often tell a woman that she needs an episiotomy to avoid prolapse of the uterus later. In all the medical literature there is no evidence for this. Or they tell her that it is safer for the baby as it prevents pressure on its head. Again there is no evidence. Healthy babies cope well with being pressed out of the vagina. It is only those already short of oxygen who need to be born quickly and who may benefit from episiotomy.

Sometimes the doctor asserts that an episiotomy is easier to suture. Maybe. But the woman might not have a tear anyway, or have one that is smaller than an episiotomy. Then there is the old myth that she will suffer less discomfort after an episiotomy and intercourse is less likely to be painful afterwards.

Jenny Sleep's study, done in a teaching hospital where standards of care are good, showed that there was no difference in postpartum perineal pain between those who had episiotomies and those who had stitched tears. But where stitching is not done well the sideways angle of the cut may make healing more difficult. When a woman tears she tends to do so straight down towards her anus. There is a natural division between the muscles there, so stitches do not pull as much and stitching is easier.

The study also showed that nearly 20 per cent of all mothers wet their pants three months after the birth. This suggests that there is something about the way labour is managed, especially when the baby is being pushed out, which subjects muscles and ligaments to great stress. Questioning the practice of episiotomy should be part of bigger questions about why women are told to push and hold their breath and strain to get the baby out, within a time limit set by the hospital. Conducting the second stage of labour as if it were a prize fight, with the woman battling against her own body to get the baby down through the barriers of flesh, causes bruising and tearing that has long-term as well as immediate effects.

Whether or not a woman needs an episiotomy has a lot to do with the position in which she gives birth. The incidence of perineal tears is highest among women who are tethered in the lithotomy position.[55] Lying flat on her back with her legs in the air puts the tissues around the vagina under great strain. Yet it became a normal position in the West because it was an easy one in which doctors could deliver babies. An obstetrician in Brazil, Dr Paciornick, was a pioneer of squatting for delivery, as women have done all over the world since time immemorial. He made an astonishing film of squatting births in which the tissues around each woman's vagina could be seen fanning out like an accordion and the babies seemed to ooze out. Dr Michel Odent, who believes that in birth the woman needs to trust her instincts, thinks that a standing squat may be the best position (and that it makes any complicated delivery, such as a breech birth, safer too.) He performs an episiotomy on only eight per cent of women. There is evidence from eight randomised controlled trials involving 11,651 women in hospitals in six countries that a warm compress placed over the perineum in the second stage of labour helps protect it.[56]

Midwives often take it for granted that women will have perineal pain after childbirth. Some mothers say a midwife or doctor asked them, 'What do you expect after having a baby?' or told them not to make 'a fuss'. But more and more women wonder why it is necessary to be damaged by birth. Some use their right to refuse an episiotomy. In law, an episiotomy that a woman has been subjected to without her consent is assault and battery. Pregnant women are taking practical steps to reduce the likelihood of a cut being needed, or a tear occurring, by improving the tone and control of their internal musculature, learning consciously to relax the vagina, prepare the perineum through regular massage with oils, and 'breathe' the baby out slowly.

Relationship counsellors see couples who, because the woman has been badly sutured, are still having sexual problems a year or more after the birth. Sometimes she has been told by a doctor that everything is anatomically normal and it is implied, if not actually stated, that it must be all in her mind. Occasionally sessions with a psychotherapist are advised. There is no doubt that having your genitals cut and then stitched up is likely to produce a strong emotional reaction. It would be the same for any man who had a surgical cut made in his penis.

After the birth the woman may no longer be able to bear penetration. She is too sore or tender, especially if her partner goes in for rough and rapid intercourse. This is *not* because she is neurotic. It hurts! A doctor's 'It's all in the mind' approach ignores and trivialises what she is saying. It is rather like things that are sometimes said to women with morning sickness, 'You must be rejecting the baby', or to those with painful periods, 'You can't accept your femininity.' In the same way, sexual problems after episiotomy are dismissed and it is suggested that they are somehow the woman's own fault. Increasingly women are refusing to accept the burden of guilt that this kind of diagnosis places on them. Pain after being cut and stitched is real.

Throughout the West we are shocked by the suffering caused to many African women by female circumcision – the slicing out of the clitoris and sewing up the labia so that there is only a small space for urine and blood to pass through. Television has shown us the horrors of clitoridectomy and infibulation. We ought to look more critically at our Western culture of childbirth and see what that does to women, too. If a cut isn't medically necessary, why are so many women's sexual organs surgically incised and then stitched up again? Episiotomy is our Western ritual of female genital mutilation.

Episiotomy does not prevent severe lacerations, because when a woman is pushing deliberately under instruction her episiotomy is often extended into a third- or fourth-degree laceration. One study revealed that when episiotomy was performed the perineum was nine times more likely to rip open.[57]

Yet episiotomies are still performed as part of the normal management of labour in the western culture of childbirth. Until recently some hospitals in Europe and the USA had close on 100 per cent rates.

After examining and evaluating numerous studies of episiotomy the UK National Institute of Health and Clinical Excellence (NICE) concluded that 'there is considerable high-level evidence that the routine use of episiotomy ... is not of benefit to women either in the short or longer term, compared with restricted use',[58] and a Cochrane review commented, 'Restrictive episiotomy policies appear to have a number of benefits compared to policies based on routine episiotomy. There is less ... suturing and fewer complications, no difference for most pain measures, and severe vaginal or perineum trauma.'[59]

Even when there is shoulder dystocia (ie, one of the baby's shoulders gets stuck) an episiotomy may do more harm than good. In one year 94,842 births at Brigham and Women's Hospital in Boston, Massachusetts, were reviewed, during which the episiotomy rate dropped from 40 per cent to four per cent and there was no change in the rate of episiotomy necessary with a shoulder dystocia.[60]

7

BIRTH AND LANGUAGE

The language of birth is never value-free. It reveals how we think about birth. But more than this, it *shapes* the way we think about it, too. Language both mirrors and defines experience.

The Great Goddess

The split between motherhood and sexuality dates from the time when patriarchal religion conquered worship of the Great Goddess. Gerda Lerner analyses it this way:

> 'My thesis is that, just as the development of plow agriculture, coinciding with increasing militarism, brought major changes in kinship and gender relations, so did the development of strong kingships and of archaic states bring changes in religious beliefs and symbols. The observable pattern is: first, the demotion of the Mother-Goddess figure and the ascendance and later dominance of her male consort/son; then his merging with a storm-god into a male Creator-God, who heads the pantheon of gods and goddesses. Wherever such changes occur, the power of creation and of fertility is transferred from the Goddess to the God.'[61]

Mary the mother of Christ was a virgin. She represents purity. She is different from all the goddesses of pagan religion. When two midwives visited her in the stable after the birth they were amazed to discover that her hymen had not been broken. Jesus was conceived in the spirit, not the flesh. The Mother Goddess embodied sex as well as power and love.[62]

Patriarchal cultures isolate sexuality from tenderness and nurture. Sex became part of male omnipotence – expressed in the way men look at women, the language they use about them, and the acts they perform on them. Perhaps this is why any connection between sexual feelings and giving birth seems bizarre to many women. Some accept spiritual language and use it to express how they feel about birth. But sexual language is dismissed as crude, a claim to a superior birth experience that is not only false but degrades other women for whom the memory of birth is dominated by sheer pain. They have recourse to male language to describe how birth is, and often to the language of obstetrics. This shapes women's perception of the experience they have lived through as a physical and emotional ordeal and a terrifying crisis.

In obstetric language birth is an equation between 'the three Ps' – the pelvis, the powers and the passenger. The mother is invisible. Her beliefs, emotions, the social context in which she lives, her relationships, her psychosexual experience – and her brain – are missing. Labour is perceived as if it occurred in a machine that either works, fails to function, or starts to work and then stalls. When doctors and midwives describe pregnancy as 'high risk', a pelvis as 'untried' or 'inadequate', a cervix 'incompetent' or labour 'prolonged', talk about 'failure to progress' – and make casual comments about a 'lazy uterus', a 'sloppy cervix', or a 'boggy fundus', they impose a view of the female body as a machine always at risk of breaking down.

In 1903 J Whitridge Williams published the first edition of his classic *Obstetrics*. The frontispiece was an illustration explained as 'Vertical Medial Section Through Body of Woman Dying in Labour, with Unruptured Membranes Protruding From Vulva.' The core of obstetrics was established – and has remained – as pathology.

We can only imagine what happened in the delivery room as this dying woman presented such a splendid opportunity for obstetric illustration: 'Get the camera on to it! Find the right angle! Hold on! Shoot a couple more!' It is an obscene photograph.

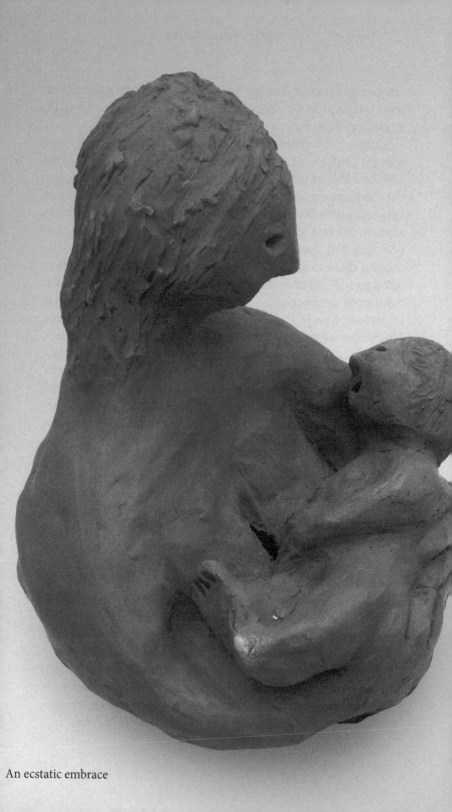

An ecstatic embrace

The baby, placenta and umbilical cord are called 'the products of conception'. Birth is described as if it were an industrial process.

Robbie Pfeufer Kahn has made a detailed analysis of the many editions of Williams' *Obstetrics* in *Bearing Meaning: The Language of Birth*.[63] It went through 17 editions until 1985 – six of those in his lifetime – and more than 100,000 copies have been sold. In it we can see how the medical system has appropriated the language of birth. It goes back a long way.

Kahn shows how Williams consolidated medical power in the USA, helped to destroy midwifery, and was responsible for the move from home to hospital birth 'so that medical students could have hands-on experience'. Starting with the 15th edition, all illustrations of normal birth were deleted.

He was dismissive of women in medicine and his lectures were scattered with Rabelaisian anecdotes 'completely disdainful' that there was a scattering of female students in his audience. It was as if they did not exist.

Kahn writes that in the 15th, 16th and 17th editions the word 'midwife' is eliminated from the index, though 'Midwifery, history of' is quoted in the 18th edition. In fact, it is about the history of forceps. This was at a time in the USA when the profession of nurse-midwifery appeared, together with a new kind of lay midwife.

Hospitalisation is explained as the reason why mortality rates in childbirth drop. Kahn writes that some of the countries in which hospital birth is the norm and those with the most obstetricians have among the highest mortality rates – for example, Israel.[64] She writes that rather than being an assembly line, in fact hospital birth is a 'disassembly line', in that the product is not put together but taken apart. [65]

Caesarean section equates the obstetrician with God. He 'caused a deep sleep to fall upon Adam, . . . took one of his ribs, and closed up the flesh instead thereof'.[66] Williams' pronouncements constitute the definitive statement of American obstetrics.

Williams removed birth from the organic cycle of life and replaced it with birth 'from above' to turn it into an industrial process. 'The only known potential of the uterus, other than to house products of conception, is to harbor disease.'[67] Hysterectomy is the grand finale of the de-creation story of birth.

Joseph DeLee taught generations of medical students in Chicago in the 1920s that routine episiotomy and forceps delivery was the only safe method to avoid disastrous damage to the mother and brain injury to the baby. Without it, children would grow up to become psychopaths and criminals.[68] He wrote that birth is a 'pathologic' process: 'If a woman falls on a pitchfork, and drives it through her perineum, we call that pathological – abnormal, but if a large baby is driven through the pelvic floor, we say that it is natural, and therefore normal. If a baby were to have its head caught in a door very lightly, but enough to cause cerebral hemorrhage, we would say that it is decidedly pathologic, but when a baby's head is crushed against a tight pelvic floor, and a hemorrhage in the brain kill it, we call this normal ... In both cases, the cause of damage, the fall on the pitchfork, and the crushing of the door, is pathogenic ...' He then moves from farm to fisheries: '... I have often wondered whether Nature did not deliberately intend women should be used up in the process of reproduction, in a manner analogous to that of the salmon, which dies after spawning?'[69]

Much obstetric language is derived from conflict and warfare. The pelvis is an arena in which a battle for survival is fought out. The fetus 'competes' with the woman for nutrients, threatening her as its head grows larger, and in labour forces its way through muscles and tissues, damaging bladder, urethra, anal sphincter and perineum.

One doctor opened a talk to pregnant women with, 'If you make a sagittal section of a corpse of a woman who died in childbirth you will see . . .'[70] Discussion of the pelvic floor muscles after childbirth was introduced with, 'Your vagina, which will have been greatly stretched during the birth, will never again return to its prebirth dimension and women were warned to avoid baths in the last months of pregnancy 'as this may damage the vagina'.[71] I remember my own GP examining me in late pregnancy and remarking, 'I think I can feel two heads' instead of suggesting that she thought there were two babies there. A physiotherapist friend recalls with horror how she used to talk about the fetal head 'hitting' the perineum.

In the language of neo-Darwinism: 'The scene is set for a competition between the fetus and the mother. It is inappropriate to see human labour as a harmonious process . . . Rather than indulging in reflex pleas to "return to the simplicity of nature" (which is often "red in tooth and claw"), we should be concentrating on making Caesarean section even safer.' This ignores social and environmental aspects of birth. In the 1920s Professor Solly Zuckerman studied baboons in London Zoo and said that they lived in a perpetual state of violence. Other researchers could not replicate his findings when working with baboons in the wild. It turned out that baboons in the zoo behaved like this because they were in captivity.[72] And, of course, there is 'delivery'. Post is delivered, milk is delivered. In a human context delivery implies salvation by a superior being.

Today buzzwords in maternity care can be deceptive. '*Continuity*' is one. In a hospital where there is a policy of one-to-one midwifery 20 women were video-recorded through labour.[73] One hundred and eight professional caregivers went in and out of the room during these labours. Midwives sat and talked to women only 15% of the time. No doctor ever sat down and had a conversation with a mother. In spite of lip-service to continuity of care, for most women it was fragmented.

Another buzzword is 'choice'. Women are told that they should make 'informed choices'. 'Informed refusal' is rarely mentioned. Better communication is the basis of choice. But communication is seen as a way of getting compliance. A psychologist writes, 'There are numerous benefits to improving communication. When these are utilised, not only satisfaction, but successful recall, compliance and informed consent can be increased.'[74]

Even so, not all obstetricians are happy to spend time listening to women. An obstetrician once snapped at me that he couldn't stand 'back seat drivers'. He meant women who had ideas about what they wanted in childbirth.

Some obstetricians are willing to spend time talking to their patients, though they may be happier giving advice, explanations and reassurance than listening to them. Indeed, one obstetrician in a major teaching hospital where one in four women had a Caesarean was pleased that there is 'increasing maternal input into childbirth'. It is not clear what he means by this. Women have always had a lot of 'maternal input'. Doctors could not produce babies without them.

The rhetoric of 'choice' ignores the pressure exerted on women to have a particular birth place – hospital – and kind of care – obstetric management, and the power of the medical system, so that discussions about choice often amount to emotional blackmail.

The concept of '*control*' in birth has changed radically over the years. When the Lamaze method was introduced in the 1960s it was self-control by a woman who used the right 'pain-prevention techniques'. Marjorie Karmel's *Thank you, Dr. Lamaze* promoted the exercise of systematic and honed reflexes, rigid training in breathing and 'differential relaxation'.[75] The woman should be able to tense up a leg or arm while keeping the rest of her body 'decontracted'. An achievement, perhaps, but not one that has direct relevance to labour. It only succeeded if she could record the birth as 'painless'. At delivery, as one woman put it, 'The obstetrician was the conductor; I was the first violin.' Lamaze warned that 'intellectual people' were less likely to succeed than working class women. 'Intellectual conceit meant that a woman was "certain to fail".'[76] An obstetrician in Moscow spoke proudly to me about the success of the training there: 'The labour wards are silent now. The mothers make no sound.' The hospital had gained control over women, who no longer disturbed the orderly running of the wards. At the Clinique des Metallurgiques in Paris, where Fernand Lamaze introduced psychoprophylaxis, when I was stopped in my tracks by a woman screaming, the obstetrician said, 'Oh, ignore her! She did not do her exercises properly' and ushered me on. I returned and asked if I might sit with her. I told her that I had five children myself. She became calm, and relaxed into her breathing. I did not criticise her but offered her silent support, and she gave birth smoothly and joyfully.

In Britain 'choice' is often presented as just a matter of opting for an elective Caesarean or vaginal birth, an epidural or self-hypnosis, and such. In a restaurant, you look at the menu, and decide that you will have a risotto or the pasta. But birth is not like that.

It is not enough to use the language of choice and women's rights. We need to find a metaphorical language for the psychosexual experience of birth. Birth is like huge tidal waves, the sweep of the wind, the cycles of night and day, and the spinning of the planets. We need to explore what it is that makes a woman free to let creative forces sweep through her. How does it feel when we are in control? It is to be free to let go. Empowerment is not something that one person can hand to another. What does it mean to be empowered? And how are women disempowered?

A midwife with the Albany Midwifery Practice in Peckham, South London, that was subsequently closed down, was ordered to attend an assertiveness training course so that she could guide women to 'correct' choices. Midwives who support women in their own free choices are more at risk of being reported to the Nursing and Midwifery Council and losing their registration.[77]

Some teachers talk about techniques for handling labour as 'weapons' and the birth as 'B-D day', implying that birth is a battle which has to be won, certainly not a psychosexual process.

A textbook on obstetrics states that the woman must 'force down' and contract her abdominal muscles, whilst bracing herself against a solid object. 'She pulls on the handbars and at the same time bears down as hard, and for as long a period, as she can. With each contraction the pressure on the perineum and rectum stimulates the patient to move towards the head of the table and out of the best position. Shoulder braces will prevent this ... At the stage where the head is passing through the introitus the patient has the sensation of being torn apart.'[78]

In French psychoprophylaxis they talk about 'verbal asepsis', and say it is as important as physical asepsis. But even that is a negative concept, suggesting keeping anxiety-producing stimuli at bay instead of using language creatively.[79]

With psychoprophylaxis, breathing exercises proliferated and as I travelled on lecture tours across the United States and in Canada and the UK I was often asked if I taught 'Huff and puff, slump and blow, choo-choo breathing, the sigh, levels A, B, C and D, H out, Hoo-hoo, Sssss, tune-tapping' or whatever else. I wonder if the mothers were as confused as I was. It tended to be very noisy, and labour wards hummed with activity as women breathed their way through contractions, often to the dismay of midwives who saw these exercises as rites which were exhausting for mothers and midwives alike.[80] All this added to the complete de-sexing of childbirth.

Books marketed to pregnant women often echo or repeat medical birth language. A well-established best-selling book in the USA warns against home birth because there are no 'facilities for an emergency cesarean or resuscitation of the newborn'.[81] Low-risk women who insist on a home birth should make sure that 'a fully equipped ambulance is standing by, ready to transport', 'at a moment's notice'. The phrase 'if it is allowed' is constantly repeated. In labour a woman can suck ice cubes or sip fluids only 'if it is allowed'. A traumatic birth is attributed, among other things, to 'thinking about and expecting pain' and 'self-pity'.

My first book, *The Experience of Childbirth*, published back in the 1960s, stimulated a flood of letters from women finding words for their experience, often for the first time.[82] Ever since then women have written to me, rang, and later e-mailed, striving to put into words their joy and often their ecstasy. Others tell of distress caused by caregivers who treated them like 'meat on the table' or 'fish on a slab'.[83] They seize on the word '*pain*'. Only when they use the language of pain do other people accept their suffering. They talk about *time*, too, because the listener is more likely to acknowledge the ordeal when they stress the length of time they had to endure pain.

Yet in women's language the important element always emerges as the relationship with their caregivers. When they say they are told 'I had to' or 'I wouldn't be allowed to', when 'they spoke about me, not to me', or 'told me it was my fault because I didn't push hard enough', birth is traumatic.[84] Where the language they use reveals a positive mutual relationship even a difficult birth is triumphant.

Birth as Rape

Women who suffer traumatic births use the same language as victims of rape.

Two of my daughters were working on Rape Crisis help lines and we talked about what they were learning from women. Over the same time women often rang me to talk about birth experiences – happy, sometimes ecstatic, ones, and others that were traumatic. As we compared our work it became clear that women who were distressed after birth used the same language as survivors of rape. They spoke about shame and disgust with themselves and their bodies, about guilt that they had in some way caused the violence, and how they felt different from other women, and isolated. They were haunted by similar images of being trapped, overpowered, physically assaulted and mutilated, and had flashbacks, nightmares and panic attacks.

They put me up in the stirrups and everything and I kept trying to close my legs, and they kept opening my legs up, and they're touching me and wiping me. You can feel them pulling and pushing at you, and I kept pushing them away.

Linda was a teacher and said she could control a class of rowdy 14 year olds. She told me that she was normally assertive and confident. She examined options, and weighed up pros and cons before coming to a decision. Now she felt that her self-confidence was destroyed completely and she had become a different person, whom she despised:

The birth of my baby was horrendous. I feel I was violated. I can't face going back to the hospital to talk to anyone there about it. I can't even drive past the hospital without breaking out into a sweat . . . I have nightmares and flashbacks to the birth, as if it were happening all over again. I feel I haven't any control over anything.

I started the Birth Crisis Network to provide effective listening for women who had reached the point – sometimes months or years later – when they felt able to talk about the experience with someone who understood and accepted, held back on giving advice, and enabled them to discover within themselves the power to handle what they were going through – somehow come to terms with it, and move forward.

This is different from 'debriefing', which suggests to me a brisk trot through a patient's case notes, explaining to her why interventions occurred and why they were justified, with the implication that she should be grateful because they were done for the sake of the baby. Yes, perhaps. But *she* matters, too, and the effect on her may have been catastrophic.

It is also different from dishing out advice about how a woman can put it behind her and get on with her life, an injunction often repeated by friends and family who long for her to stop talking about her trauma and be positive and constructive, because she should be glad she has a healthy baby.

When birth is experienced as institutionalised rape you are supposed to thank the very people who violated you. A woman is then in a double-bind, caught between horror and gratitude.

Anyone who suffers post-traumatic stress after childbirth (PTSD) cannot just switch it off. It goes round and round in her mind like an endless video. Acute memories, flashbacks to events, intense sensory experiences involving physical contact, being stuck in positions when she was poked and examined, sounds of people's voices and radio programmes in the background perhaps, smells of hospital disinfectant and the curry the midwives were eating along the corridor. These come rushing back, often to overwhelm her when she least expects them – and at night. Turning on the TV to find a birth scene confronting her, driving past the hospital, or encountering one of the midwives at the supermarket checkout – all these may bring flashbacks and panic attacks.

For, like a soldier who served in Vietnam or Iraq, she has been imprinted with the details of vivid events in which all control was taken from her. To give birth was as if she was trapped in a machine and spat out at the other end with a baby.

Psychological research suggests that 1:20 women suffer PTSD after birth. But, as with rape, many cases are hidden from the statistics, because women feel they are not justified in going to the doctor, or they do and are diagnosed as depressed – and treated with anti-depressants. In fact, they are in a state of heightened anxiety and panic, which is different from depression. Those who are labelled as depressed may become depressed the longer they remain in this state of red alert.

Any change in the way we perceive ourselves affects relationships, too. A male partner may be traumatised, as well. He felt he colluded in this act of violence. He blames himself for not intervening. She may blame him for the same reasons. He cannot bear listening to her talking about it any more, so he switches on the TV, flings himself into work, goes off to the pub with his mates, or simply ignores her. They drift further and further apart. A woman who has had an episiotomy that has extended into a laceration (which is how most severe tears occur), who may have been badly sutured so that for weeks she feels she is sitting on jagged shards of glass, or one who suffers bladder and bowel incontinence, is unlikely to enjoy sex for months – or years.

Melissa, the mother of a two year old told me:

They decided on a trial of forceps. I told them, 'Please try and tell me what is going on.' The man who seemed to be in charge said, 'Are you a doctor? Mind your own business!' I felt like I was being attacked.
I went to my GP afterwards because I needed to talk about it. I felt I had been assaulted. And I was still so sore down there making love was out of the question. He told me I had psychosexual problems and that I was depressed. I said, 'I am not depressed. I am bloody mad!'
I don't know where to turn for help.

A woman may feel as if her baby does not belong to her. This is more likely after an emergency Caesarean section. When her baby girl was born Felicity had forceps and a large episiotomy. With an epidural in place, she didn't have pain. She said:

I didn't feel a thing. My experience left me disconnected from her. During pregnancy I felt as if I knew every inch of her...When she was born I did not feel as if I could identify with her.

Or a woman may feel that she is not 'really' a mother, but goes through the motions and tries to behave like one. She may even secretly blame the baby for the way the birth turned out. Or she protests that she 'loves him to bits' and hopes that the mother-baby bond will somehow compensate for her trauma.

Birth does not have to be like this. No woman should have to look back on it as rape. We should respect research evidence that reveals that many interventions that have become more or less routine either bring no benefit or are actually harmful, including automatic induction of labour when a woman goes ten days or a week past her due date and continuous electronic fetal monitoring.[85] Yet research in Canada shows that it takes on average 15 years before such evidence changes practice. Obstetricians often proffer the threat of litigation as the reason why they advise an elective Caesarean, induction or continuous monitoring. It is 'just in case' obstetrics, and may explain why only 47 per cent of births in England are listed as 'normal'. One-to-one midwife care through pregnancy, birth and the days after is a major factor in preventing unnecessary Caesarean sections.

Every woman also needs the opportunity to make informed choices and to create her own setting for birth, whether that is in a hospital, birth centre or at home, outdoors or indoors, on dry land or in water and with or without family, other supporters or one special birth companion. In these ways we could humanise our culture of birth. We could transform birth from an act of rape to one of fulfilment and joy for both caregivers and mothers everywhere.

In the same way that genital sex can be abusive or life affirming and exultant, birth can be thrilling and intensely pleasurable or leave a woman feeling cheated, trapped and raped.[86]

The Making of an Obstetrician

How do obstetricians learn? And what do they learn?

The Royal College of Obstetricians has remodelled its training as part of a programme called 'Modernising Medical Careers'. With 1,500 consultants in obstetrics and gynaecology, the plan was to create 1,000 more consultant posts. These upper echelon obstetricians/gynaecologists were to work in larger units and have fresh opportunities to specialise. Drawing on reports from the Royal College of Obstetricians and Gynaecologists[87,88] two clinical lecturers writing in the *British Medical Journal* list these skills as:

Assisted reproduction
Management of infertile couples
Maternal medicine
Menopause
Preparing for obstetric leadership on the labour ward
Ultrasound imaging in gynaecological conditions
Urodynamics
Medical education
Fetal medicine

In spite of the fact that the RCOG reports state that the purpose of reforms is to offer improved care, the *BMJ* paper does not contain a single reference to women.

A budding obstetrician's personal qualities are described this way:

'The ability to adapt to rapidly changing situations is essential, and a sense of humour is useful when you are faced with difficult situations. Enthusiasm, agility, and an intention to enjoy life are key features for this role . . . If you want a challenge, excitement, and an adrenaline rush, but also a fulfilling career, look no further than obstetrics and gynaecology.'[89]

The focus of the obstetrician is on intervention, management, technology and surgery.

I think they have got it wrong. Midwifery is much older than obstetrics, and, yes, dealing with and averting emergencies must be exciting, but the care of women in pregnancy and childbirth is much more than that, and defining this care as obstetrics leads to interventions that inevitably prove iatrogenic.

Women need midwives. But they also need obstetricians who acknowledge and understand midwifery skills, and who learn from midwives.

One great advantage of the traditional system of obstetric training in Britain is that medical students and interns learn from watching and working alongside experienced midwives. This is how they get an idea of how to keep birth normal. Every caregiver should know how to give unobtrusive emotional support, respect the natural rhythms of labour and birth, and hold back. Far from seeking an adrenaline rush, he or she needs to be able to 'centre down' and honour the physiological process.

This can only happen when midwives have the autonomy, sensitivity and self-confidence which comes with continuity of care, and when there is one-to-one midwifery that enables the midwife to develop a relationship with each woman through pregnancy, birth and post partum. When midwives work in this way they teach budding obstetricians precious skills.

I have observed midwives working with women in many different cultures and see that they often have to protect women from obstetricians, their adrenaline rush, and what the authors of that article call the 'Red Savina Habanero' (the world's hottest chilli pepper) of medicine. The successful obstetrician seems to be an adrenaline junkie.

Some obstetric teachers are aware that there is little to do with women in the formal syllabus, and invite a National Childbirth Trust teacher in to give a talk to their students. The Royal College of Obstetricians and Gynaecologists now has a regular slot on birth trauma in its education programme. When I address students on these courses I note that many of those participating are working for the first time in the UK. The authors of the *BMJ* article have some special tips for them: 'Getting informed consent may be an unfamiliar task, so practise some mock scenarios with your friends'. (It is not clear why their friends should be best for this task, but it is better than nothing. And there is no mention of informed *refusal* and what an obstetrician should do about that).

Some senior lecturers teach communication skills. This is often limited to learning how to clarify, explain and elicit a positive response to proposed interventions.

Others are more imaginative, but meet institutional resistance. When a lecturer in obstetrics in a London hospital had medical students act being pregnant women in an antenatal clinic students objected vehemently. They refused to have their legs raised and spread apart in lithotomy stirrups. They said they felt 'humiliated'. Instead of using this to gain some insight into how women feel, the experiment was axed.

I met a woman who thanked me for being instrumental in setting her son on a fulfilling obstetric career path. This was a surprise. I speak in schools occasionally, to pupils of any age. She reminded me that I had been invited to lecture about birth to the pre-university class at a prestigious boys' public school. I arrived with my baby doll and foam rubber vagina and acted giving birth, pushing and breathing as the tissues of the vulva fanned out, and demonstrating the thrill and sexual arousal of an undirected spontaneous second stage in which the woman responds to the waves of power and elemental desire sweeping through her body. I had been anxious that the privileged youths sitting in the front row, legs spread wide, hands in their pockets, supercilious, even sneering, expressions on their faces, would think I was a mad woman. But I gave my all.

This young man decided there and then that he wanted to be an obstetrician, and was now fully qualified. I wonder how often he had the opportunity to see a normal second stage. But at least he knew what it could be like. Most obstetricians don't. They don't realise that getting a woman into an alien environment, kick-starting labour, clock-watching dilatation of the cervix and descent of the presenting part, putting her up on a delivery table, harpooning her to a fetal monitor, watching her critically, fixing her legs in stirrups and telling her to hold her breath and push as hard and as often as she can – all these are interventions that make birth abnormal.

We should bring drama into obstetric education – theatre, role play (not just with friends, but including childbearing women who can teach from their own experiences) and conversation analysis of real-life talking. Communication skills are still dealt with at a level that might be suitable for training laundry detergent salesmen, but not caregivers in childbirth. Role play, drama, comedy, and women's personal accounts of experiences are valuable tools to teach understanding and develop skills in communication. Obstetricians need to know how to turn a baby from breech to vertex, how to tackle haemorrhage, and perform a Caesarean section. But there is more to obstetrics than that. Episiotomy and suturing of the perineum, for example, is not only a question of why, when and how, but of the effects that surgical genital mutilation and subsequent repair can have on women's feelings about their bodies, their self-esteem, their sex lives, their relationship with a partner, and with the baby.

Conversation analysis is deconstruction not only of subject matter, but of pauses, breaths in and out, intonation, inflexion, and the sounds we make that convey understanding, surprise, sympathy, and validation of what a woman is saying. It is about listening reflectively and responding, about the flow of a relationship, not just how to put over ideas and get the client on your side.[90, 91]

Conversation analysis could enrich and add a new dimension to obstetric education and reflective practice.

Obstetric education should not be only about the management of childbirth and medical and surgical interventions, but also the obstetrician's role in interacting with women, and increasing awareness and understanding of this.

What Do We Tell Our Children?

Our gut feelings about birth are conveyed to children even when we are unaware of it, and certainly are not doing so intentionally.

Joy in birth is infectious. But so is fear. The words we choose matter, our facial expressions, even sounds that are not deliberate. Hushed conversations intended to shut children out indicate a topic is taboo. And our reactions to birth scenes on TV send out clear messages.

Children start to learn about birth long before any formal education starts, and years before they are exposed to formal sex education.

When adults think of birth as a painful ordeal, this is what children learn from us. When we think of it as an exciting adventure it opens up the possibility that they come to see it as an intense psychosexual experience in which the power of a woman's body brings new life.

As they grow older, too, analysis of the workings of institutions and medical systems is one element in asking searching questions about society.

Part of the work we did when my daughter Celia and I researched our book *Talking with Children About Things that Matter*, thanks to a grant enabling us to have special time writing in Belagio, was learning from children's drawings about sex and birth.[92]

Midwives in the Czech Republic asked school children all over the country to let them have pictures of babies being born. The result was a superb collection which they gave to me for analysis. Pictures from ten year olds fell naturally into home birth scenes in which children shared the experience and had been present at the birth and hospital scenes where children drew on their imagination and invariably delivery was an horrendous event, the abused mother manacled, her legs in lithotomy stirrups, and exhibited like a lab specimen under bright lights with her torturers leaning over her and poking and cutting. In the home birth scenes the family was participating and eagerly reaching out to hold and cuddle the newborn, bringing food and drinks for the mother, nestled together on the bed, smiling and laughing. The contrast was dramatic. Nobody had given these children lessons in how birth could be a happy psychosexual experience. They knew it because they had lived through and shared the love and excitement in the family. The others drew in great detail scenes of activity like those on a conveyor belt of capture, imprisonment and torture similar to those in their comics which depicted struggles between 'goodies' and 'baddies'.

We can't offer children a pristine representation of birth. They are likely to pick up on pain and brutality from TV and the internet, from those whispered conversations 'not in front of the children', stories spread in the playground, and the contagious fear expressed or disguised by adults. But we can send positive messages about the joy of birth and the energy that sweeps through the mother's body. That is quite different from 'sex ed' in the classroom.

Manufactured and artificial stories of uplift and light are unlikely to convince children either. They see through the pretence. If an experience has been distressing we need to understand why, and how birth can be made an ordeal, with women left feeling trapped, helpless, cheated, complete failures, guilty and sexually abused. The way we give birth is a human rights issue. This is how children can begin to understand the politics of birth and other institutionalised relations between those in power and those who are subjected to it.

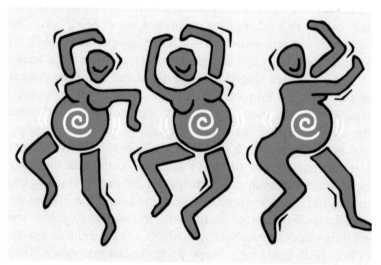

Zumbabump: Movement and dance before, during and after pregnancy with baby too.

8

BIRTH DANCE

A pregnancy yoga teacher, Nadia Raafat, writes: 'Pelvic circles in figures of eight help to disperse the pain and assist the baby in finding the optimal fetal position for entry of the birth canal. The movements also produce a soothing rhythmic effect that alleviates discomfort and promotes a healthy unfolding of the labour process.'

Medical anthropologist and founder of Birthlight Dr Françoise Freedman claims that the 'camel walk' where the woman undulates her abdomen, helps prevent a baby from getting into a posterior position.

Nadia Raafat goes on to say that during pregnancy, 'Belly dancing offers a raft of health benefits: pelvic and lower abdominal movements send additional blood flow to female organs, enhancing growth and healthy functioning of the body; the basic posture, with the knees slightly bent and the tailbone tucked under, is excellent for correcting spinal misalignment, relieving lower backache; and like yoga, belly dancing leads to increased strength and flexibility, both of which are important during labour.' She goes on to describe dancing on the floor, where the woman gets onto her knees and does back bends. 'She sinks to the floor drawing strength from the earth as she advances through the later stages of labour.'[93, 94]

Breathing Awareness for Labour

There are three simple breathing exercises to explore as you move your body freely, and imagine breathing through a contraction in labour. After each choose one of the suggested resting positions.

1. Exhale slowly through your mouth so that you can hear the sound. Pause briefly at the end of each breath, and then inhale slowly through your nose. Continue for three to five cycles of the breathing rhythm, and relax.
2. Breathe as in exercise 1 and focus awareness on the contact your body is making with the ground. Breathe the pain away into the earth each time you breathe out, and then let the breath flow in again slowly. Again, continue for three to five cycles of the breathing rhythm, and relax.
3. Using the techniques of exercise 1 and 2, experiment with making low level vowel sounds as you exhale. Try 'oooooh' and 'aaaaah', releasing the sound from deep inside. Many women find that expressing sounds freely in labour helps to reduce pain. As the contraction peaks let your breathing speed up. Keep it light as a feather. As the contraction fades breathe slowly and fully. Continue with three to five cycles of the breathing rhythm, and relax.

Start as soon as the imaginary contraction begins, focusing on the out breaths and 'breathing pain away': I suggest that you move into a quicker, lighter rhythm over the peak of the contraction if this feels right. Otherwise continue breathing fully and slowly. Then relax for a while, using one of the resting positions suggested at the end of each exercise. Let go of your body and allow your mind to drift. Breathe spontaneously and easily, in and out through your nose. As the contractions get stronger you may find you need to make more noise as you are breathing out. If so do it triumphantly and loudly! This will help you release and let go of the pain. Be aware of the earth underneath you and stay 'grounded' through the contraction.

In the weeks approaching birth, practise every day for just five to ten minutes, combining position, movements and breathing.

When labour starts, wait as long as possible until in established labour before you swing into a dance. When contractions become so strong that you need to focus entirely on them combine the breathing with dance movements.

Resting Positions

Resting using a chair
- Sit on a chair, knees apart and lean forwards, resting your upper body on a table or desk.
- Place a pillow over the back of a chair, and sit astride the chair, leaning over the pillow.

Kneeling resting positions with upper body support
- This time put the pillow on the seat of a chair in front of you. Kneel letting the pillow take the weight of your upper body.
- Relax over a beanbag so that your upper body is completely supported.

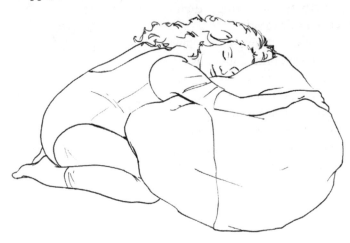

Resting positions kneeling or squatting with your whole body supported
- Kneel forwards onto a beanbag or pile of large cushions so that your whole body is supported.

• Squat supported on a stool, leaning forwards.

Kneeling Upright Dance

In this vertical position gravity will help the contractions to be more effective. Use it in labour if you still have quite a long way to go, as an alternative to standing. This position can also be used in a birth pool.

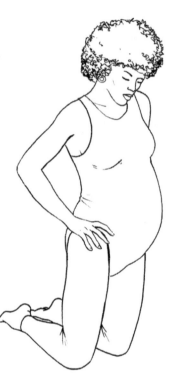

• Kneel on the floor on a soft surface with your knees slightly apart. Relax your arms and shoulders and rest your hands on your hips, letting them hang loosely by your sides or holding on to a support.

• Roll your hips, making soft, circular movements, or alternatively swing them from side to side.

• Breathe through a few practice contractions, using the breathing awareness exercises, and then relax.

• You may spend a long time kneeling in labour, so protect your knees by placing soft pillows or a foam mat under them.

Half Kneel/Half Squat Dance

It may be helpful to use this as a variation on kneeling positions from time to time during labour. Many women enjoy it and find it helps to relieve pain.

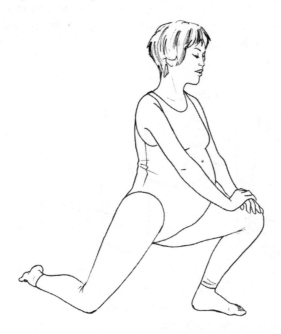

- Begin in a kneeling upright position on a soft surface. Lift one leg with the knee bent and the foot on the floor.
- Relax your shoulders and arms, placing your hands on your bent knee.
- Breathe out, and lunge gently forwards towards the bent knee.
- Breathe in, and come back slowly to the more upright starting position.
- Repeat this movement four to five times. Change legs and repeat on the other side. Then relax.

Kneeling on All Fours

Kneeling on all fours feels very secure, offering support from the ground and helping you avoid distractions as you focus on contractions. Horizontal kneeling can help during the rapidly recurring and intense contractions at the end of the first stage, and if you have a backache labour, it will encourage a baby in a posterior position to turn into an easier anterior position by the time you move to the pushing stage.

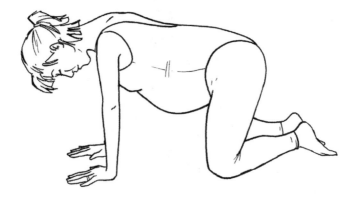

- Kneel on a soft surface on the ground, palms down in line with your knees. It may be comfortable in labour to place a small cushion under each ankle.
- Relax your neck and shoulders, and feel the weight of your head. Breathe evenly and feel the way your hands and knees are in contact with the floor.
- Roll your hips, making soft circular movements. Now swing your hips from side to side, switching weight from one leg to the other in a smooth movement.
- Work through the breathing awareness exercises while moving in this position, and then relax completely.

Rocking

When kneeling on all fours in labour it can help to rock your body forwards and backwards with your hands on the ground. Move slowly and avoid arching your lower back as you come forwards.

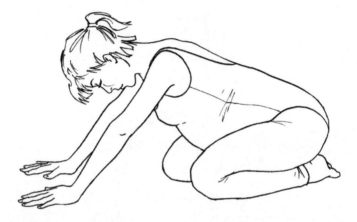

- Kneel on a soft surface on the floor on hands and knees. Your knees should be comfortably apart. Focus awareness on your breathing and on the contact your body is making with the ground.
- As you breathe in, bring your weight forwards onto your hands without arching your back.
- Breathe out and swing your pelvis back towards your heels.
- Repeat these movements five or six times, rocking forwards on the in breath and back on the out breath, and then relax.
- Now try rocking movements using the breathing awareness exercises.

Standing Dance

Standing up and moving your pelvis during contractions helps encourage the progress of labour. Leaning forwards as you move will ease the pain and help position your baby head down, with the back of the head at the front. Relax in between contractions.

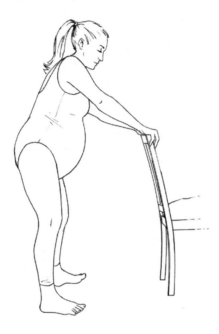

- Stand with feet well grounded and comfortably apart so that your whole body feels loose.
- Hold onto the back of a chair and bend your knees, rolling your hips slowly, making easy circular movements. Then try swinging your hips slowly from side to side.
- Imagine a contraction and breathe through it using the breathing awareness exercises, and then relax.

Belly Dancing with Your Unborn Baby

Maha Al Musa's descriptions of traditional Arab belly dancing in pregnancy and birth were inspiring – I have learned a lot from her.[95] The belly dance expresses the power of women to produce life. It is about connecting with the source of female sexuality.

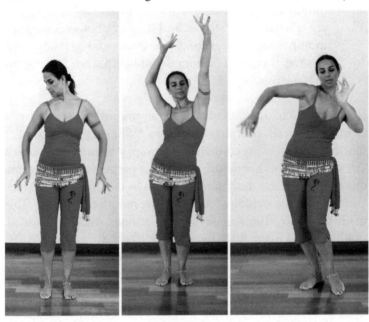

- With your torso naked (wearing a bra if you like) or in a nightdress or loose smock, slip a large head sash round your hips. A long silk one would be splendid or any lightweight scarf. A fine tablecloth, a runner or tea towel will do. You may be able to come up with a jewelled or chained belt to loop on your hips. The more whatever you wear helps you feel flexible, the more light-hearted you can be.
- Massage the baby in the cradle of the pelvis with gentle, loving hands. Then start rolling and rocking your hips in response to the rhythm. Keep it as smooth and sensuous as you can. It is a way of showing love for your baby.

- Feel what happens inside and the way the muscles contract and release.
- Switch on some evocative music. Explore how you and the music link in the dance.
- Be aware of what is happening in the muscles of your face, too, especially in and around your mouth. When your mouth is relaxed the muscles in and around your vagina are relaxed, too. In the second stage of labour release your mouth instead of gritting your teeth and pressing your lips together. Sing or hum if you like. Surrender yourself to the sensations.

Ina May Gaskin, the famous American midwife and 'mother of all midwives', calls contractions 'rushes'.[96] She suggests to couples that they kiss, drawing on their sexual energy, as each rush comes. The woman opens her mouth around her partner's lips. Kathleen, one of the mothers describing her birth in the book, says: 'Mark and I started smooching a lot to keep my mouth really loose. This made the contractions come on really strong.' And Mark added, 'Kathleen had never kissed me before like that . . . I could feel electricity coming out of her nipples. It was like touching the end of an electrical terminal.'

Some of the exercises I include have been adapted from those taught by Janet Balaskas, who was a student of mine, training to be an NCT teacher, and who created the Active Birth Movement that revolutionised antenatal education that had previously been based first on Dick-Read and then on Lamaze teaching.[97]

9

WATER BIRTH AND SONG

It is sometimes claimed that water birth has a long ancestry and that labour in water occurs in a variety of cultures. There is little anthropological evidence for this. Women have usually sought out, or have had built for them, a secluded, dark place, a room by the stove in temperate climates, a fern-cushioned space in the bush, a mossy enclosure, or a sand- or fern-carpeted tent.

There is a Maori mountain tribe where women give birth in a sacred river. Some Polynesian islanders went down to the beach to give birth, where they could have a dip and freshen up immediately afterwards. But in general water has been in short supply and too precious to be used for birth. Like eating the placenta, water birth is more likely to have been developed in recent times in California than in traditional cultures. Water birth is part of a new birth culture that challenges the dominant medical system of birth. It does not need to be validated by tradition.

Women luxuriate in water during labour and often want to stay in the pool for birth. Sometimes this is an ordinary household bath. But a problem with a bath is that the sides are often narrow so that the mother cannot move easily. It may be difficult to have the water deep enough to cover her lower torso. Instead, she is sitting in a puddle.

When floating in a pool, a woman in labour can move unencumbered. The water bears some of her weight and she has a feeling of being in her own private world within the margins of her pool. The water enables her to move spontaneously. She squats, kneels, lies on her side, goes on all fours, or crouches forward holding on to the side of the pool.

She explores gliding movements, using her arms to move forwards and backwards during contractions and to turn from her back to one side, or from one side to the other, rolling her pelvis. She lunges, bending one or both knees and pushing away from the side of the pool. She rolls her knees from side to side so that she is also rolling her pelvis. She rediscovers birth postures and movements common to traditional birth cultures all over the world, in touch with her body and responding to the messages it gives her. Birth is a psychosexual experience.

Following concerns about safety, a landmark study of 4,032 babies born under water in England and Wales between April 1994 and March 1996 was undertaken, involving all consultant paediatricians in the British Isles.[98] It revealed that the perinatal mortality rate for babies born under water was 1.2 per 1000, comparable to that for low-risk babies born in air. No deaths occurred as a result of water births. Thirty-four babies were admitted to special care baby units, a rate of 8.4 per 1000. This is much lower than the rate for babies born to low-risk primigravidae.

If labour starts naturally, a woman has no drugs, and the baby is born with the cord intact into warm, fresh water; the baby does not breathe until the head surfaces into cooler, drier air. The clamping of the umbilical cord provides a further stimulus for breathing.[99]

Water birth offers a radical change in how a woman behaves, and what she is allowed to do, in labour. Most hospitals in the UK have at least one pool installed. That is the good news. In practice, pools are often not used, because they are not made readily available. A midwife excuses herself saying that she has not been 'trained' to do water births. (It is not a matter of training, but rather simple good midwifery and being happy to be 'hands off').

Or a woman may be told that the pool has not been cleaned since the last mother used it. Sometimes the junior registrar, or some other weary doctor, is sleeping in the room where it has been installed. And sometimes it is just loaded with junk! So when you finally sink into warm water it may have been after quite a struggle.

A study in one hospital based on unstructured interviews concluded that midwives did nothing to promote water birth because this did not match their priorities, which stemmed from having to rush from one woman to another and write up notes before hurrying to the next one, and institutions did nothing to back midwives who were rushed off their feet.[100] It is not only a matter of having the pool and midwives being skilled but the organisation in which the midwives worked.

'I resented being asked to get out of the water to be examined.'

When a woman is labelled as 'high risk', the pool is out of the question because the baby's heart must be monitored. This is not a good reason for being refused a pool. It is possible to record the heart with an underwater sonic aid. If that is not available a standard intermittent monitor can be slipped inside a condom to waterproof it.

Many women who have enjoyed immersion in water describe how it helped them relax. They could surrender themselves to the water and delight in its buoyancy, floating freely, letting the uterus create the birth energy, and harmonising with it as it does so. They can roll and dip, curve and arch, bend and stretch, rather like a dolphin in what feels like an effortless water dance.

A woman lunges, bending one or both knees and pushing away from the side of the pool. She rolls her knees from side to side so that she is also rolling her pelvis. She explores gliding movements, using her arms to float forwards and backwards during contractions or to turn from her back to one side, or from one side to the other, rolling her pelvis over as she does so. She rediscovers birth postures and movements common to traditional birth cultures all over the world.

The fact that the mother is in a protected space – her private territory – is one of the benefits of using a pool. Other people do not crowd in. Her caregivers are kept at arm's length – unless they are very eager to intervene. She may choose to have her partner in the water with her, but many women do not.

Birth accounts suggest that most women value the boundaries of the pool and it helps them feel safe and free to breathe and move as they wish.

'I'd choose water birth again because it reduces the pain and increases mobility.'

Pain turns into suffering when we feel trapped. Being free to move helps a woman handle contractions *her* way. She can leave the pool whenever she likes.

Women who have used a birth pool say they enjoyed being in their own space where nobody was going to push a hypodermic syringe or intravenous drip into them. They were not 'messed about', and could move freely in water. It is not a matter of getting into different positions and then being stuck in them, but of moving – gliding from one position to another, circling, unlocking and tilting the pelvis, kneeling forward and backward, and making rippling movements with the spine.

'As soon as I got into the water I felt safe, secure, free. The water cradled me. I wasn't heavy any longer – and I could move.'

The water needs to be deep enough to cover the top of the uterus if a woman is to get adequate pain relief and be able to float. It is important that her pelvis is not raised above the level of the water, since a baby who slides out into air and then gets dunked may inhale water.

'As my baby was born I wouldn't have dreamed of getting out. It would have interrupted the whole process. It would have been like saying "You must lie down on your back."'

Or perhaps it is like someone saying, just as you are about to reach orgasm, 'Hang on a moment! You can't do that here. We are going to move you now.'

The more midwives help with water births, the more they like them. They often develop an understanding of birth that is denied midwives who work in hospitals where it is the practice to hurry birth and tell women when and how to push.

When a midwife attends a water birth she should watch and wait. She does not intrude. She respects the spontaneous rhythms of labour. She learns about the normal physiology of birth in a way it is impossible to do in any hospital where active management is practised, everything must occur in a set period of time, and drugs are used to stimulate the uterus.

'I have never seen a birth like this before. The mother knew exactly what to do without being prompted.'
When a woman can focus on the power of contractions and work with them, she responds in a smoothly co-ordinated way. Instead of fighting her body, she listens to what it is telling her.

'Water births are peaceful. There is no need for commanded pushing. The mothers seem much more confident that what they are doing is right.'
An unforced second stage, with no deliberate breath-holding or straining, contributes to a psychosexual experience. A woman can follow her instincts, and the result is that she feels more in control during labour and after the birth.[101]

'The perineum is usually protected by the water. As a result an episiotomy is rarely needed.'
A woman with an intact perineum avoids the pain of stitches and feeling that she is sitting on thorns for weeks after.

A study of over 2,000 births in an unusual Swiss hospital was published in the medical journal *Fetal Diagnosis and Therapy*. In this hospital all mothers could choose between a birth stool, a wide comfortable bed, a rope hanging from the ceiling, a wheel they could grasp, and a pool. Half the women chose water birth. In a questionnaire later they marked a point on a line that went from 'dreadful' at one end to 'wonderful' at the other. After a water birth most made a mark on the line close to 'wonderful'. Those who gave birth in bed marked points further away. Those who used other methods selected points in between. The study showed that water birth is as safe as more conventional methods. Women used far fewer painkilling drugs, were less likely to need an episiotomy, or to bleed heavily, and birth was as safe for the baby as birth in air.[102]

For first-time mothers there is evidence that the place where the birth pool is has an impact on birth outcomes.

Women are better able to relax and let sexual feelings flow in a birth pool. At home or in a freestanding midwifery unit this is easier than in hospital or a midwifery unit attached to a hospital.[103]

Women having their first babies are less likely to be transferred to an obstetric unit and more give birth spontaneously.

Song

The earliest birth in water recorded in Western Europe occurred in Pithiviers, France, some time in the 1970s. Dr Michel Odent had introduced a children's paddling pool into the birth room at the little hospital there, so that a woman having a painful labour might have the benefits of submersion in water. The first water birth took him by surprise and he stepped into the pool still wearing his socks to catch the baby. In fact, the pool was so successful in easing pain, enabling women to act instinctively, and facilitating the progress of labour, that he then installed a specially designed pool. The birth pool became the hallmark of this hospital and a symbol of his philosophy of birth.

Michel and I met at a conference on psychoprophylaxis in obstetrics, which was held in Rome, at a time when I was living near Pithiviers, and he invited me to come and see what he was doing there.

In 1977 I visited the hospital. It was not with the aim of seeing a water birth. Rather, it was to explore the non-obstetric milieu for birth which he had created with a group of dedicated midwives. Pithiviers was essentially women's space, though fathers, other children and all members of the family were made welcome. As in traditional environments all over the world, birth was shaped and conducted by women. It was the same with pregnancy.

An enthusiastic older woman who had been an opera singer

gathered pregnant women, and whole families, round her piano in the antenatal clinic, and they and any members of staff who could drop in sang together unselfconsciously, rousingly and jubilantly. It was a powerful bonding experience. Singing was an important element in antenatal clinic visits.

Song in other cultures

Singing in pregnancy and birth is a well established practice with a long history in many different cultures. Women form choirs to welcome pregnancy, to guide a women through it with counsel and hope, to support her and join in the sounds she makes during labour, to praise her and greet the baby at the birth, and to announce the birth to the village.

Among the Galla of Ethiopia, for example, when the expectant mother returns to her mother's home to give birth she takes with her two, four or six women to be her companions, at least one of whom must be an accomplished singer.[104] Birth takes place in the back room of the house, and the mother kneels on freshly strewn grass, supported by her women friends. The male anthropologist who wrote about this did not describe what they sang during labour, presumably because he was not allowed to be present. But as soon as the baby is born the women ululate, four times for a girl, five for a boy. Then they break into songs which proclaim the mother's gallantry in giving birth and her happiness, and give thanks to Maram, the goddess of childbirth. They compare the mother's achievement with that of the brave hunter who returns victorious to the village.

In New Zealand, when a Maori women is pregnant a female choir traditionally sings to her about the progress of the pregnancy. If all is not well, they sing about this, too, preparing her for problems ahead. Pregnancy links women together in shared pleasure and concern which is expressed through song.

Rachel Beckett, a midwife, writes:

'The concept of using music during labour and birth is not new, but it is useful to consider the multitude of ways in which music can contribute to birth, from providing focus, to distraction from potentially disturbing external noise, improving mood, providing a sense of familiarity and control, motivating movement and, perhaps more significantly, reducing anxiety.'[105]

Why Water? Why Not Song?

It intrigues me that water birth has become an alternative birth option for increasing numbers of women, and that many hospitals have installed pools, while singing, the other important element in the Pithiviers birth style, and a much more common practice in diverse cultures, has never caught on in Britain or North America. Song can be a celebration of sexuality. Why not express joy in the sexuality and richness of birth by singing?

The problem cannot be cost. A piano is not more expensive than a birth pool. Singing is unlikely to be considered an unevaluated risk factor.

One possible answer is that the social system of the modern hospital dictates the relative status of the behaviour of everyone in it. Singing in groups would blur the boundaries between staff, and between staff and patients. It might be disturbing for those who relied on a rigid social system to define their position and role and to maintain order in a hierarchically based institution. It is difficult to imagine informal singing groups consisting of consultants, midwives, cleaners, pregnant women, children, fathers and senior managers, or a choir singing while a woman was in labour in any NHS hospital.

On the other hand, singing can be formalised, as it is in church services and temples, where chanting conforms to a strict pattern. The priest intones the collect and, with careful timing and in unison, the congregation responds. There is no doubt about who is in charge, and the worshippers must not usurp the priestly role. It is conceivable that singing might be introduced into hospitals in a similarly regulated way, and that it would then reinforce, rather than blur, the hierarchical system. So this is an unsatisfactory, or at least incomplete, explanation as to why singing does not find a place in birth today.

Water has a powerful cultural symbolism that makes it particularly attractive and there is a long tradition of using water for healing: sacred springs, spas and 'taking the waters'. It is an essential element in the Christian baptism. In revivalist sects the faithful are 'born again' by submersion in water. Water birth draws on this traditional symbolism, bestowing the birth pool with esoteric meaning.

Yet communal singing is also rooted in northern cultures. It often marks major life transitions – wedding and funeral hymns in the rites around marriage and death, for example. It has a unifying function. When people join together in a national anthem, sing '*Jerusalem*' on the last night of the Proms, or football crowds roar out songs in support of their team, or traditionally when workers have toiled in the fields, singing has cohesive power.

Consumer Choice

The dominant model of birth in northern industrial cultures today is both technocratic and individualistic. Birth is technologically managed and with electronic fetal monitoring, intravenous drips and epidural cannulae – all regulated by the clock, the oldest technology of all, on which all the other technology is based. The object of attention is the fetus in the pelvis and the patient in which the fetus is contained.

When a woman presents in an antenatal clinic, or is admitted in labour, she is 'managed' as an isolated reproductive organism, separate from her family and community. The web of relationships in her life outside the hospital doors is seen as irrelevant, or, if it intrudes, as an inconvenience to be dealt with by teaching midwives about ethnic minorities and the communication and management skills required to achieve patient compliance.

Over the last 25 years women have begun to resist being treated as ambulant pelvises and contracting uteruses. The result is that the focus is shifting, slowly but inexorably, to the 'whole woman'. But that is as far as it goes.

A patient is seen as a consumer who must be given the information to make choices between alternatives. These are ranged in front of her: induction of labour, pethidine, breathing exercises, and epidural, a 'walking' epidural, an elective Caesarean section, or water birth. The pregnant woman selects what she wants, much as she would a breakfast cereal on the supermarket shelf.

Song, in contrast, is part of a communal experience. Traditionally, in cultures throughout the world, birth is an activity shared by a group of women who come together to support the woman in labour and thereby reinforce the bonds between them.

Though in some cultures the ideal is for a woman to go off into the bush alone and come back with a baby, these societies are few and far between, and even there, a woman having her first baby is usually attended by several female friends. The norm in most cultures is for birth to draw together a group of women, all of whom already know each other well. It takes place in women's space, and is choreographed by them. Prayer and invocation, embraces, joking, the telling of stories and sharing of news in the community, sounds of encouragement, massage, movements, dance and song all have a place in the unfolding birth drama.

Groups of women singing are foreign to birth today in northern cultures. This is so because the experience of birth has been medicalised and socially fragmented.

A woman nearing the end of the pregnancy may not even know who will be attending her during labour. A group of female friends, especially if they were singing and in festive mood, would be unlikely to gain admission to the birth room. She is lucky if she has even one individual who stays with her through labour and till after the birth. If this happens, it is likely to be a male partner, perhaps with no previous experience of birth.

Childbirth is no longer an act shared between women who are well known to each other, in which the bonds between them are reinforced and celebrated. It is an isolated process which is seen increasingly as a matter of individual consumer choice. A consumer may be permitted, with careful negotiation, to opt for the use of a birth pool. If one is available it can be offered as another 'method' and incorporated into the hospital system. Singing, in contrast, does not fit the paradigm of birth 'methods' and techniques that can be regulated by agreed protocols. Perhaps this is why the other element in the birth experience at Pithiviers has still to be explored.

HOME BIRTH, MIDWIVES AND DOULAS

Home birth

In the USA home birth is part of an underground movement of mothers and midwives who resist the institutionalisation of birth. Under one per cent of births take place at home. Compare that with a rate of 30 per cent in the Netherlands.

In 2008 the American Congress of Obstetricians and Gynecologists warned its members against what it called 'trendy' home births. In spite of, or perhaps because of, its medicalised, high tech system of birth, the USA has one of the highest rates of maternal mortality in the industrialised world and the most expensive technology. Around one in three births are by Caesarean section.

A group of 13 midwives in New York practised home births but lost the right to do them in 2010, when a progressive hospital in Manhattan, St Vincent's, was closed down because of bankruptcy. The midwives who worked with it could no longer practise legally and lost the only backing they had from obstetricians, and their insurance cover.[106]

Home birth in Britain

Home birth has at last been accepted as an informed choice for women who want to avoid potentially harmful interventions and to control their own birth experience so far as they can. The change of direction was first noted in a report by the Royal College of Midwives in 2002 which observed that 'home birth can no longer be regarded as a special privilege for a fringe minority – it should be understood as integral and mainstream to any modern maternity service'.[107]

Why do Women Decide on Home Birth?

Natalie summarises her reasons for choosing a home birth by saying bluntly: '*The advantage was that I felt that I could do whatever I bloody well liked*' and she added,

> '*Home birth is all about the body and mind acting in unison, feeling safe and expressive and not acting in a way you feel you are supposed to, and required to, like good sex.*
>
> *My independent midwife totally prepared me psychologically, and gave me strength. I would feel violated, almost raped, if I went into hospital and had things done to me, put inside me etc, if I felt it was unnecessary. I wouldn't trust them either. Hospitals and Friedman's Curve are a patriarchal form of controlling women's bodies.*'

Women assert their right to a home birth because they want to reclaim the experience as intense and personal, just as good sex is.

In 2007 the UK National Institute for Health and Clinical Excellence (NICE) issued clinical guidelines on the intrapartum care of healthy women and their babies. Under 'key priorities' it stated: 'Women should be offered the choice of planning birth at home, in a midwife-led unit or in an obstetric unit . . . for women who plan to give birth at home or in a midwife-led unit there is a higher likelihood of a normal birth, with less intervention.'

Its other recommendations included: 'A woman in established labour should receive supportive one-to-one care', 'should not be left on her own except for short periods or at (her) request', and 'Clinical intervention should not be offered or advised when labour is progressing normally'. 'The opportunity to labour in water is recommended for pain relief' and 'Before choosing epidural analgesia, women should be informed about the risks and benefits, and the implications for their labour'.[108]

Soon after this came out, the Maternity Care Working Party, made up of representatives of the Royal College of Obstetricians and Gynaecologists, the Royal College of Midwives and the National Childbirth Trust, produced a consensus statement on the need to recognise, facilitate and audit normal birth.[109] What is normal? Is it simply what happens routinely to women in hospital labours? Is it the absence of interventions? If it turns out that each intervention leads to another, which are the most damaging, and which the most likely to have short or long-term harmful effects? If a specific intervention is revealed as having negative consequences, why was it deemed necessary? 'Normal' delivery includes 'women whose labour starts spontaneously, progresses spontaneously without drugs, and who give birth spontaneously'. It excludes 'induction of labour (with prostaglandins, oxytocics or ARM), epidural or spinal, general anaesthetic, forceps or ventouse, Caesarean section, or episiotomy'. It recommended: 'choice of place of birth including home birth, a midwife-led birth centre and a maternity unit with midwifery and medical facilities', and 'the chance for women to get to know their midwife prior to labour'.

Maybe home birth would not have been re-evaluated if Caesarean rates had not soared and research evidence revealed morbidity and long-term side-effects that shocked many obstetricians, not only health activists and mothers, into asking how, in a culture that attempts to regulate childbirth with prompt intervention and sophisticated technology, we have got into this mess.[110-116] John Davis, Emeritus Professor of Child Health at Cambridge University, observed: 'It is so often the unnerving atmosphere of a busy obstetric unit for a woman in labour that brings about the very problems that it is equipped to deal with.'[117] In other mammals, too, a hostile environment inhibits the hormonal surge that stimulates spontaneous behaviour and results in longer labours and perinatal deaths.[118]

Are women really 'too posh to push'? Some opt for a Caesarean because they believe it is a safe and painless way to have a baby. This is often because they have gone through ghastly vaginal births and cannot face delivering like that again.[119]

Yet records of Birth Crisis, my help-line for women trying to handle distressing birth experiences, reveal that approximately 80 per cent of women seeking help with post-traumatic stress following birth have had previous Caesareans. For them surgery is not the answer to distress. It is the cause. The knowledge that home birth is a viable option may be the only thing that enables them to start on another pregnancy, or, if they are already pregnant, to get through this one and stay sane. Rulings that home birth should only be a choice for low-risk women are irrelevant. They are willing to take the risk.

For the first time there is official recognition of the dangers of hospital birth and the advantages of birth in an environment that a woman herself controls. It may not sound like a revolution, but it could introduce one if practice follows precept.

In some ways this is putting the cart before the horse, because these changes can't happen until all midwives are educated about home birth and have personal experience of it, feel confident and don't try to bring the hospital into the home. This is not only a matter of giving women choice, but about assessing the risks and benefits of different settings for birth, the quality of relationships that are created between caregivers and the women they serve, and knowing how to set the scene for a psychosexual experience. Experience of home birth should be an essential element in all midwifery education, rather than a specialised skill for a few individual midwives and small teams.

Even so, and even when home birth is planned well ahead, it may not be an easy journey. Natalie, whom I quoted earlier, told me that with her first birth she had difficulties with the NHS midwives assigned to her:

'I had problems with the community midwives in that we had to come to a compromise about what they wanted and what I wanted. I had to draw up a birth plan which had to be approved first. When

I went into labour they refused to come out to me at first because I went into labour early one morning at the weekend. My husband and I had to argue with them. When they did come out to me I don't think they really understood what home birth was like, because they were continually surprised by my progress and quietness. They also chatted all the way through whilst I was trying to focus, which was annoying, but I zoned myself out. I could smell the cigarette smoke on them after they had gone out for a fag and came back in. My husband supported me physically whilst I birthed. They were observers.'

Heather Parker, Director of Midwifery for Torbay in Devon, where each woman can decide once she is already in labour whether she stays at home or goes into hospital, tells me that they had a 12.8 per cent home birth rate in 2006-7, which was increased by February 2007 to 18 per cent.[120]

The Albany Midwives[121] worked in an area of London that has a rich ethnic mix with many mothers from a wide variety of cultures. They did not select out low-risk groups for home birth, but served the needs of all women, who were free to choose home birth. Becky Reed says that of 210 women they attended between January and December 2006, and among whom there were three sets of twins, 46 per cent gave birth at home, 82 per cent had a spontaneous vaginal birth, 15 per cent Caesareans, and 3 per cent ventouse or forceps. 93.6 per cent of the women who gave birth spontaneously had no analgesia and 19 per cent gave birth in water. 70 per cent had an intact perineum, and there were no episiotomies at all. 73.5 per cent had a physiological third stage. 78.8 per cent were breastfeeding exclusively at 28 days.[122] Sadly, King's College Hospital, of which the Albany was a part, closed it down.

In the UK hospital midwives are leaving the profession because they are frustrated, subject to institutional bullying and punitive treatment, and feel trapped on the conveyor belt of a task-oriented, rather than a woman-centred, system of childbirth management. As I talk to midwives who assist at home births regularly, it is evident that their work, in contrast, is not just rewarding, but that midwives and mothers share a unique and precious life-enhancing experience.[123]

Midwives

A woman's relationship with her midwife is central to her experience of birth.

Research reveals that the quality of this relationship is the single most important factor in being able to look back on the birth as a satisfying experience.[124,125]

This is a major element in *The New Midwifery: Science and Sensitivity in Practice*, a ground-breaking book about the need for every midwife to have up-to-date knowledge of birth-related research, and also to work with emotional and social aspects of birth.[126] Each midwife needs the skills and sensitivity to meld the art and science of midwifery.

Lesley Page suggests five steps that need to be taken for evidence-based midwifery:

1. Finding out what is important to the woman and her family; providing personal care requires that we understand the values, anxieties, hopes and dreams of the woman expecting a baby . . . It is of paramount importance that the issue of safety is not used to restrict women's choices or their ability to be in control of decisions.
2. Using information from the clinical examination;
3. Seeking and assessing information to inform decisions;
4. Talking it through;
5. Reflecting on outcomes, feelings and consequences.

Research I undertook in a major English teaching hospital showed that it is often difficult for a woman to get to know her midwife and for a midwife to get to know the woman for whom she is caring.[127, 128]

Women who are cared for by a number of different midwives whom they never get to know say they felt 'confused' and 'bewildered'. They lose confidence. Many feel 'abandoned': *I was disappointed that the first midwife had to go off-shift and leave 50 minutes before the baby was delivered, as I had built up trust in her and had a rapport with her. I didn't have the opportunity to do this with M ... in the second stage of labour.'* Another woman, who had a previous still-birth said: *'One midwife who knew my history might have made a great difference. They were complete strangers. You ought to know your midwife.'* I found that women who never got to know the names of their midwives had a more negative experience of birth than those who had named midwives, particularly when they had five or more midwives. Those with a positive experience usually knew the names of their midwives and said: *'It was great to have the midwife as my friend';* *'The positive experience was dependent on having the midwife of my choice who I had built a relationship with and had confidence in. This can be very hit and miss depending on who was on call. I was lucky.'*

A midwife is unable to give focused care if she has to rush from one patient to another and rely on an epidural and an electronic fetal monitor to take her place. Women said: *'We had one midwife covering four women, all close to delivery';* *'I was left alone for 35 minutes plus while being monitored in the admission room. By the time the midwife returned I was nine centimetres dilated.'* One woman said that every time another midwife appeared on the scene she did a vaginal examination: *'It was the worst and most traumatic aspect of the birth.'* Women also remarked on how midwives did not share information when they handed over to somebody else. So they had to tell the midwife their priorities, if there was time, and they had the courage to do so, to each different midwife.

Women had to relate to a number of 'team members'. *'The room felt like Clapham Junction with people bursting in and out and a ward round coming in unannounced';* *'There was a constant stream of registrars, consultants, house officers, anaesthetists and students in and out of the room all of the time';* *'I felt desperately the victim of lack of communication. There were too many people.'*

Even women who had a positive birth experience in hospital were appalled at conditions on postnatal wards: *'All I ever kept hearing was, "Oh, sorry, we are just too busy at the moment"'.* They had very little help with breastfeeding, and many received conflicting advice, *'I found it very confusing to have different advice from a huge number of midwives*'; '*I never saw the same midwife twice*'. Some women were discharged with breastfeeding not yet established, their self-esteem very low, and feeling in one woman's words, '*totally exhausted*'.

When a continuing relationship with a warm and understanding midwife is positive in pregnancy, right through labour and birth, and in the hours after, and the midwife holds back and leaves space for the mother to respond spontaneously to the rush of hormones in her bloodstream, birth and the transition to motherhood can be a profound psychosexual experience.

In many Eastern European countries women's health issues are submerged by political and economic crises, home birth has been criminalised, midwives are forbidden to attend them, and women must give birth in often squalid conditions in unsanitary and decrepit hospital wards where even basic hygiene is difficult. The rhythms of spontaneous birth are managed and distorted in such a way that women experience birth as rape.

Responding to this challenge, the European Network of Childbirth Associations, ENCA, was founded in 1993, as a network of individuals and consumer organisations campaigning for improvements in perinatal care for mothers and babies. Representatives from nine countries joined at first, and later fifteen member organisations: Austria, Bosnia-Herzegovina, the Czech Republic, Germany, Greece, Hungary, Italy, Luxembourg, the Netherlands, Poland, Slovakia, Switzerland, the UK and, more recently, Latvia and Russia. They meet in a different European country each year. Members respond to appeals for help from childbirth organisations and circulate research so that these countries can challenge medical orthodoxy.

I had already started to study what was happening in the ex-Soviet countries of Eastern Europe and lectured at conferences organised by activist groups unhappy about the denial of women's autonomy in childbirth.

In some European countries there are way too many obstetricians. I have visited Italian maternity units where there are fewer midwives than doctors. Italian midwives were ordered not to attend home births, too, and must restrict their role as community midwives to pre-partum and postnatal care of mother and baby. The majority have not resisted this. When presented with protocols for care produced by obstetricians their only way to protest is to falsify records, so that, for example, women making slow progress in the second stage are recorded on the partogram as having a much shorter expulsive stage than actually occurred. Midwives are trapped in a system they dare not try to change.

In the north of Italy and in Spain, however, small groups of midwives bravely got together to improve care and offer women choices such as home birth. But in challenging the institutional system they, like midwives in the US, put their careers at risk.

This is the dominant theme in Hungary. In April 2008, at the invitation of Ágnes Geréb and the Alternatal Foundation, I went to Budapest to lecture on Home Birth Day, and this included talks to midwives, home birth parents and a wider public. Halls were crowded with eager audiences, including professionals, and my book, *Birth Crisis*, was translated and published to coincide with this. Events were filmed to be used for further publicity and as a basis for wider discussion.

Since 2007 independent midwives there have been harassed by the Board of Obstetrics and face media persecution. Because they were forbidden to assist at home births they re-invented themselves as doulas who accompany women into hospital, but do not 'deliver' babies.[129] A new alliance between parents and those professionals who are critical of the present system has developed, too, striving for 'non-institutional' and 'free' birth.

Doulas

Doulas are the modern equivalent of godsibs, traditional birth sisters and friends who came to support a woman when she went into labour.

The Standards of Practice of DONA International, the US-based doula association, are explicit about interaction between doulas and professionals in the health service: 'The doula advocates for the client's wishes as expressed in her birth plan, in prenatal conversations, and intrapartum discussion, by encouraging her client to ask questions of her caregiver and to express her preferences and concerns.' She 'enhances the communication between client and caregiver. ... the advocacy role does not include the doula speaking on behalf of the client or making decisions for the client. The advocacy role is best described as support, information, and mediation or negotiation.'[130]

In the UK the doula movement is strong, and women in Holloway, the largest women's prison in Europe, can choose a birth companion, too.[131,132] Many doulas have been midwives or become doulas as a step towards midwifery training. Adela Stockton, who was herself a midwife writes, 'We protect her birth environment, we support her partner to enjoy his/her new baby being born, we nurture the new family. Doula work should not be misconstrued as "backdoor midwifery"'.[133,134] The Doula Code of Practice states that a doula offers support, but not advice, exploring options and enabling the woman to make her own decisions 'wherever and however she chooses to give birth – home/birth centre/hospital, with or without medical interventions, whilst a postnatal doula supports the mother whether breast or bottle feeding'.

She 'does not perform clinical or medical tasks, diagnose medical conditions or give medical advice, even if trained as a health professional prior to becoming/whilst working as a doula'. If she is 'qualified as a therapist in some other field and wishes to apply this skill in her practice, it must be made clear that they are two separate roles'. She 'will refer clients to other appropriate resources/professionals should the clients have needs beyond the scope of the doula role'.

A postnatal doula gives practical and moral support to a woman and her family. She helps with breastfeeding as well as housework and enables the mother to care for herself as well as the baby and helps look after older children. She is usually employed for two to four hours a day for three to eight weeks.

Doulas 'show integrity and respect at all times towards their clients, doula colleagues and other professionals with whom they may be working' and 'will not discuss personal and confidential information which has been disclosed to them by their clients … without the express permission of those clients'.[135]

If a woman giving birth to her first baby has a doula, labour is shorter by two hours on average. She is less at risk of having oxytocin augmentation and a forceps or ventouse delivery. Her body works more naturally and she can relax and enjoy the sexual energy that streams through her.

She is less likely to ask for pain-relieving drugs. The pain is not threatening in the way it is if she feels herself a victim – she is much more likely to take it in her stride and use it positively. The epidural rate is eight per cent compared with 55 per cent without a doula. Having a doula decreases the chance of a Caesarean by more than 50 per cent. With support from a doula a partner who is present gains confidence. Having a doula also increases success with breastfeeding.[136]

Jamaica

Looking back on it after many years, I realise that when I was in Jamaica and observing labours and births both in the public maternity hospital in Kingston and in the community, I was serving as a doula. My research included births at home and those in the threatening setting of a hospital in which women were treated like animals that were out of control, and the midwives – who had been trained in Canada or England – tried to shut them up and physically constrain their energy.

The mothers dreaded going into hospital and their behaviour there was in marked contrast to that in home births attended by a *nana*, the traditional midwife in the West Indies.[137]

Women drew on religion to express their torment and passion, shook, lunged, shuddered, rolled, twisted, rocked their pelvises, threw themselves around, chanted and screamed to the Lord, beseeching salvation, exactly as they did in the gatherings of the Holy Rollers up in the hills.

I was an observer, but found it impossible not to participate.

I told each woman whom I was with that I had five children and reached out to touch her firmly and hold her, but not to restrain her. When she started pushing I climbed onto the delivery table where she was forced to lie flat on her back and supported her with my body, cradling her in my arms as I had seen women do – the family members and neighbours – in rural parts of the island, so that she could be at least semi-upright.

I did not talk or attempt to change her behaviour. Her panic was always replaced immediately by co-ordinated bearing down interspersed with rest between contractions just as it was in home births in Western countries with one-to-one midwife care. I do not know how many babies were given the name 'Sheila', but quite a few, and it was clear that this sisterly support helped them come back into their bodies in a satisfying way and enjoy the intense feelings as the babies descended, their heads crowned, and then slipped out. They greeted sacro-iliac pain in a very positive way, because they believed that a gate had to open low in the spine for the baby to be born, and this was a sign that it was happening.

Since then I have been a birth companion to many women who have been in my antenatal classes who didn't have a partner, or whose partner did not want to be there, or who was willing to attend, but only to watch.

France

Midwives in France reacted to a highly centralised obstetric authority that maintains firm control over midwifery practice by responding to the doula movement in a very different way from those in Britain. They often feel trapped and their resentment and anger is directed against doulas, who they perceive as invading their territory. The Ordre des Sages-Femmes (the French equivalent of the Royal College of Midwives) accused doulas of being a religious sect which they compared with scientology – corrupting women's minds, dictating their behaviour, and engaging in arcane rites. In 2007 a press release from the Agence Française de Presse reported, 'Sects have changed their strategies, no more mystical gurus, instead tutors, therapists or lobbyists fitting into the décor without any exterior signs of proselytism, stated the Miviludes in its 4th annual report published last Wednesday'. (The Miviludes is an official inter-ministerial commission) ... 'The report went on to cite the doula training course of labour/birth companion'.[138] It is reminiscent of McCarthyism in the USA when Communists were seen lurking everywhere.

The Doulas de France responded: 'Doulas offer non medical support to women, parents from all ethnic, religious, social backgrounds, respecting their choices, wishes, religion, beliefs and *only when the pregnancy/labour is followed by a doctor/ midwife or obstetrician* and without any proselytism... Doulas de France is an "association de loi 1901" (non-profit making organisation), with a college of 8 co-chairs working with a team of volunteers, with a membership of 150 . . . Our role is a social and human one and we do not practise medical acts. We are not therapists. We aim at creating family links as well as local ones, to facilitate communication between the different health professionals and partners.'[139]

Mavis Kirkham, former Professor of Midwifery at Sheffield Hallam University, testified that in the UK doulas have a positive role to play in health care and are not a sect:

> I have maintained a clinical practice as a midwife since 1971. During that time my observations have supported the vast body of research which demonstrates the positive clinical outcomes of support for childbearing women.
>
> There is a shortage of midwives in this country and midwives are increasingly occupied with their growing technological workload. The vital work of providing continuous support in labour, therefore, increasingly falls to doulas.
>
> I have worked with a number of doulas and always been impressed with their skill, knowledge and warmth.
>
> They are used in this area to support women from deprived backgrounds, where clinical outcomes are likely to be worrying. This is done through Sure Start programmes with very good results.

Doulas are also used to improve breastfeeding rates.

Doulas give support in such a way as to enhance women's confidence and self-esteem. Thus they nurture women's autonomy and capacity to mother their babies. They also support fathers and help families cherish their new baby. This work is the exact opposite of that of sects, which seek to undermine personal autonomy and separate people from their families.

Since as a midwife I have received much support from doulas, I am shocked to hear that French doulas are seen as a sect. The work of doulas is healthy and socially positive. I see them as colleagues and wish to support them.[140]

French doulas are still at risk. Valerie Dupin tells me that the Ordre des Sages-Femmes refuses to meet with them, though there is now a doula course (in response to their demand for training.) She adds that sometimes they get calls from distressed hospital midwives who need to talk about difficulties with obstetricians and poor working conditions. They met with a member of the Ministry of Health in 2008 who had not read the dossier they submitted and dismissed any need for doulas.

'The doula team is working well together. They dance a seamless dance, caring for the labouring woman, each in their own way, with different (and sometimes the same) tasks, each respecting the others relationship to the woman and her partner, knowing when to take an active role, when to melt into the background, when to be in the driving seat, and when to be a passenger.

It is a shared birth space, with all players taking an important part, but taking their lead from the birthing woman . . .'[141]

Those who respect women's autonomy – obstetricians, midwives and doulas – need to work together to challenge authoritarianism, routine interventions of all kinds, rigidity of thinking and practice, and dogmatism.

11

SEX AFTER THE BABY COMES

Sexual adjustment is part of the wider emotional adjustments to changed social and family relationships which new parents need to make. With the birth of each baby the form of the family changes, and all the relationships of those in it are shifted – sometimes abruptly, sometimes almost imperceptibly.

Concepts of Pollution

Traditionally, in societies over the world, the new mother is fed special foods, given attention, and may be confined in a darkened room where she is kept guarded from spiritual, magic or evil influences. She and the baby are passing through a transitional state of existence.

A taboo on intercourse has the same function. The mother is told that she will get 'infected' or that 'it will open up wounds'. Even in Western societies the prohibition varies, so that whereas American women may be instructed by their obstetricians not to have intercourse for six weeks, French women are more likely to be told *'pas de rapports'* for three weeks! While some women are happy to have intercourse just a few days after birth, most are only able to enjoy it several weeks after that, especially if they have had an episiotomy and suturing of the perineum.

Tiredness

Tiredness is a major challenge. A new mother puts a great deal of energy into this unaccustomed task. She and her partner may be exhausted because of insufficient sleep, with the baby waking two or three times in the night. Tiredness is often made more intense by anxiety about caring for the baby and uncertainty as to whether she is doing it right. This combination of exhaustion and anxiety may mean that she never gets aroused because she cannot surrender herself to erotic sensations, or she falls asleep before anything much has happened. Many couples say that as they approach the end of the first year after birth they are having intercourse less often than before the pregnancy – or sometimes not at all.

One way of coping with tiredness is to start by analysing your day on paper. Plan urgent work right after breakfast. Decide what you can skip. Spend any spare money (if you have it) on household help, labour-saving machines, or if you are working from home, secretarial help. Find spaces in the day. Every baby sleeps sometimes. Plan the largest space for a rest time – in bed (with a hot water bottle or electric blanket already switched on if necessary). Take a drink on a tray and a book or magazine, or have the TV opposite the bed.

Depression

A woman may be not only tired and irritable but also depressed – and guilty because she is depressed. She is nervous about handling the baby – fearing she will drown or drop him. Or she may switch off completely. No amount of being told to pull herself together helps.

Social isolation, overcrowding, financial insecurity and poverty, these are all associated with depression, one symptom of which is loss of interest in sex.

Pain

If she had an episiotomy the skin is pulled tight and 'prickles'. After a week or so it may feel as if there is a bump of tissue which is especially tender. It is likely to be at the base of the vagina, near the anus. Any pressure against these sensitive spots is painful. If she tightens up when her partner tries to penetrate, this causes further pain. The lining of the vagina may be dry and taut. Sometimes the natural lubrication which moistens the vaginal wall during sexual intercourse does not return for a while, and extra lubrication in the form of a cream or jelly (for example a contraceptive cream or one sold for keeping the nipples soft) is necessary. Her partner can gently stroke this in before he attempts entry, and she can put a little on his penis too.

If she has been sutured, they could try a position in which the penis presses against the front part of the vagina and the clitoris, not the tender area at the back. She helps him inside so that she does not feel the need to recoil, like a snail drawing in its horns. As he slides in she releases her pelvic floor muscles so that they are suspended downwards like a heavy hammock.

Delicate and tender stimulation of the clitoris is vital. She may associate an accustomed position with gynaecological examination, so cannot be aroused in one which she enjoyed in the past.

Her lover should not press on her full breasts, as they are sensitive, particularly at night when the baby is probably sleeping for longer periods.

One of the most dramatic changes that can occur in a woman's body comes with the birth of a baby. Before, she was full. Now, empty. There was another living being inside her. Once the baby is outside there is someone who she needs to get to know and care for. During labour the body has been like the stage on which a drama has been played, or for some women, more like a battlefield. She may feel tender and aching all over – soft, open and terribly vulnerable. Women tell me they feel '*fat, leaky, tired*', '*lost*', '*fragile*', '*as though my femininity has been taken away*', '*like an old woman*', '*mess*', '*overweight*', and even, for one who revelled in having the baby inside her, *'let down because I miss being pregnant'*.

The new mother may feel like this even after a straightforward labour. If the birth has been difficult she may be frightened of and alienated from her body, and alarmed by the changes that have been forced on it. *'I felt I might tear open at any moment'*; *'After the poking and prodding I wanted time to recover and have my body to myself again.'* She may wonder if she may ever feel that her body is hers to experience with sexual delight. She may be in pain, stiff, bruised and sore, and when she shifts from one buttock to the other stitches in her perineum make her think that she is sitting on embedded thorns or slithers of glass.

It is not surprising that birth can profoundly affect a woman's feelings about sex. But it is not only a matter of whether labour has been easy or difficult, short or long and drawn out. Fundamental to how she feels about her body is the way in which it has been treated by those caring for her. If she has been treated as a person, her body handled with consideration, has been kept fully informed about what is happening, and been able to share in the decisions made about her care; she will have retained her autonomy. Her body still belongs to her and she probably feels that she has used it in an exciting and splendid way. But if she has been processed through labour as if on a conveyor belt, with little or no choice about what happens, if she was probed and treated roughly and treated as the object of a medical exercise, rather than as a person going through an experience of deep emotional significance, she is likely to feel at first that her body no longer belongs to her, but to the hospital, and later to find it very difficult to express herself through her body without inhibitions. She holds herself rigid, guarding her body from pain, invasion and injury. It can be a long journey to get her on good terms with her body after such an alienating experience, and allow sexual passion to sweep through every pore.

In the first weeks after childbirth she may be bleeding as if she had a heavy period. Her pads stick to skin which may have been nicked and just tender because her pubic hair has been shaved and is now beginning to grow again. Many women start out on motherhood feeling strangers to their bodies. Jo, for example, had a forceps delivery and says, '*I was devastated by the birth. My body felt so abused. My vagina, stitched back together, was black with bruising and I couldn't sit down. It didn't seem like my body. I didn't recognise it as mine. Sex was unthinkable. I completely retreated into myself. Whenever my husband touched my vagina I immediately thought of the birth, the doctors, the examinations, and got very upset.*'

It is not only that so many things have already happened to the mother, but that further changes take place in the six weeks or so after birth. The uterus is contracting and returning to its previous pre-pregnancy position and size. She loses the body fluids she stored in late pregnancy, partly from her bladder, but most of all through her skin in the form of sweat. She feels hot, smelly and sticky. Breasts start to lactate and get heavy and swollen, with veins like ribbons with tributaries etched all over them. They ache and are tender and milk oozes or spurts from her nipples. Before feeds she may feel that both breasts are blown up like balloons about to burst, and after they are sagging and empty.

When the main flow of bleeding has reduced it changes from brown to pink, and then is merely a clear discharge. Some women feel dirty through this time, as if all their body orifices are open and leaking, and the flow of fluids represents a kind of puerperal incontinence. No wonder they hate their bodies, and think they are ugly and soiled.

Moira says that long after the soreness and bruising had disappeared she continued to feel like this. It was because her image seemed inextricably linked with her memories of her mother, who had died when she was nine, '*She was extremely large, overweight and looked far more than 37 at the time of the death. Probably an exaggerated image, but an utterly unsexy pattern of motherhood.*'

Other women feel quite differently about this new softness and openness. Even the odour of blood may be exciting and the capacity to produce milk abundantly and unexpectedly seems like a miracle: '*My body felt delicious*', one woman told me, '*comforting, sensual, sexy, but not orgasmic*'. It may be a matter of feeling back in shape again, the kind of shape you feel you were meant to be. '*I felt great about my body after birth*', Vicky says, '*because the bump was gone and my stomach was flat again*'. For Marion, '*I felt in touch with natural forces – more sensually and sexually aware.*' It seemed for her a mystical experience, ecstatic and religious.

Some women feel a flood of vitality which they want to express even in the first days after delivery. One woman told me she hated being separated from her husband during the 48 hours after birth because she was feeling so sexy: '*The birth amazed me. I was proud that my body could produce my lovely baby. How nature can work! Afterward I felt like running around a baseball field! I was amazed how quickly my body returned to normal. I couldn't wait to get back home to my husband – and bed! I was very horny!*'

For some women the six to eight weeks after birth is one in which they feel an entirely new sense of harmony between mind and body, an astonished awareness of biological power, and what amounts to reverence for the energy and precise patterning of natural forces in the female body. There is a sense of triumph and something that I can only describe as physical radiance. Birth has been life-enhancing. There are women who even experience a natural state of languorous satisfaction like that felt after orgasm. It is as if the body has been gathered into waves of passion in labour and is now like a boat tossed on a peaceful beach after a storm.

Birth can affect men in this way, too. If they were not only present at the birth, but shared in preparation for it and were fully involved, they may become more aware of the subtleties and intricacy of a woman's body and have gained a new understanding of female sexuality. John told me that Helen went for several weeks after birth when she felt 'unclean' and very 'clinical' and said, '*I felt it didn't really belong to the "me" that I knew from before.*' But John's love and pleasure in her made her feel different. He had been there right through the birth and says he felt a deep awe for all that her body could do, and was suffused with love and tenderness for her. Before the baby came he had been a rather aggressive, high-speed lover. But after he became gentle and caring, and for the first time Helen experienced orgasm during intercourse.

There are women who say that the experience of birth has brought them to the point where they can surrender conscious control of their bodies and begin to enjoy orgasm, sometimes for the very first time. Others attribute this to the partner's changed attitudes and new tenderness. Whatever the cause, it is not unusual for women to find that sexual experience has a new depth and diversity, though some months often pass before they realise this.

Contraception

Doctors do not usually prescribe contraceptives until after the postnatal examination, which may be scheduled four to eight weeks post partum. But you do not rely on breastfeeding as a contraceptive. A man can use a condom, and if the woman is dry and tender, a spermicidal lubricant can be used with the condom. Oral contraception is not a good idea since it entails introducing drugs into your bloodstream and your milk.

Interruptions

As soon as you start to make love the baby wants to be fed. One woman wrote, *'Every time we start to have sex it seems the baby cries and then I can't concentrate, even if I know she has just been fed. I worry that something is wrong. And if she gets suddenly quiet I worry that she's died. So I don't get excited.'*

In the first few months of life the mother's capacity to respond immediately to her baby's needs is an important element in the survival of the species. Winnicott called it 'primary maternal preoccupation'.[142] It lasts at least eight to ten weeks after the birth, and for some women much longer.

One reason why a baby cries just as a couple begin to make love is that the feed may have been rushed. Get ready for going to bed and create the atmosphere you like well before the late feed so that you have ample time to spend with the baby first. Then put the baby in another room close by, or behind a screen, where you cannot hear every little sniffle and grunt. Turn on the radio or TV low, or leave a loudly ticking clock next to the baby. Babies sleep better with a regular background of repetitive sound than in total silence. Even the whirr of a fan heater can help you concentrate on your body instead of being distracted by the baby's movements, breathing and other noises.

Most new babies find it very difficult to pass between states of waking and sleeping and back again and cry as they drop off to sleep or wake up. A baby often makes restless movements or cries out suddenly 10 to 20 minutes after being put down. This does not mean the baby has colic or needs feeding. An anxious mother picks her baby up then, so preventing him or her from falling asleep.

Pelvic Floor Muscles

A figure of eight of muscle fibres surrounds the vagina and urethra in the front and the anus at the back, and supports the uterus and the bladder. When these muscles are tightened you can stop the passage of urine or faeces. You can also use them in lovemaking either consciously or unconsciously. Since they contain many nerve-endings which record pleasurable stimuli, their activity is vital for sexual satisfaction.

The clitoris is sometimes talked about as if it alone were the source of all sexual delight. Yet when a woman responds with pleasure because her clitoris is stimulated, these inner layers of muscles become active, and contract rhythmically, leading to orgasm. Sometimes a woman never achieves climax because the muscles deep inside have not been drawn into the activity.

The most important way to increase the tone and vitality of the pelvic floor is to consciously and regularly exercise it, alternatively tightening and releasing the muscles and 'talking' with them, rather as we can with muscles around our mouths, always finishing with a tightening-up movement rather than a flop and a sag. There is no need to cross your ankles or do anything with your knees, upper legs or buttocks.

Start doing this after the birth as soon as you can feel what you are doing with the perineum – to the point of discomfort, but not beyond it. Perineal tissues are often bruised after childbirth, even if you have not had stitches. Muscle is rather like a soapy sponge in bath water. The more you squeeze and release the sponge, the sooner the soapy liquid flows out and fresh water comes in. If you think of bruised muscle as like a sponge the holes of which are filled with stale blood, you will realise that the more you squeeze it the quicker will the de-oxygenated blood be expelled, and fresh, oxygenated blood will come in, promoting healing.

These muscles together form the pelvic floor. Because the pelvic floor muscles are composed of strata extending up to support the uterus and the bladder, they are not really like a floor at all, but more like a lift inside, which can go up further and further as the muscles are tightened.

Imagine that you are usually at the ground floor and you are going to bring the muscles up from floor to floor of a five-storey building. Tighten a bit and you are on the second floor. Hold them firmly there. Now go up to the third floor and hold. You will feel the pressure against your bladder, especially if it is full. Make sure you are not holding your breath. Now proceed to the fourth floor and wait a little. Finally pull the muscles up inside right up to the fifth floor. As you do this press your shoulders down to ensure you are not tightening them as you draw up the invisible muscles inside. Now your lift goes down, and you will need to proceed by very small steps. Control the muscles so they do not simply collapse to the basement. When you reach the ground floor, go up one floor again, so you finish with a toning movement.

It is a good idea to do the lift exercise every time you change a nappy, whenever you wash dishes, and wait for a bus or at the checkout in the supermarket. Always complete each cycle of movement with a slow, smooth tightening-up action.

Some women picture themselves as stretched and sagging. In the first six months after birth it is normal to notice some spreading and fanning out of tissues in the outer third of the vagina. Sometimes pelvic floor muscles are extremely slack after a difficult birth. This may occur when the woman is urged to push harder and harder and to continue doing so for a long time, and after a forceps delivery. Sagging can also occur if you get a bad cough, are constipated and strain on the lavatory, or, since the pelvic floor registers and expresses moods like the muscles of our faces, if you are depressed.

When the pelvic floor has lost its natural tone it feels as though the uterus is slipping its moorings. A woman gets low backache and feels weary. Damaged tissues can be sutured.

If your pelvic floor is very weak you may find it easier to practise these movements with your legs raised, so that your bladder and uterus are tipped back by gravity and are not pressing on the stretched hammock of muscle. One way of doing it is to lie with your lower legs raised and resting on a chair. Place your hand over your perineum and you can feel the movements underneath. When you are in bed introduce two fingers into the vagina and grip them with the muscles about half way up inside. If the muscle begins to tremble, release it and intersperse the tightenings with rest periods, as trembling is a sign that it is subjected to too much stress.

Good pelvic floor tone will probably take at least eight weeks of regular exercise to achieve.

Transition to Parenthood

Though birth is the dramatic climax of pregnancy, it is only the beginning of a host of other changes which take place both in the relationship between a woman and her newborn baby and between a couple as lovers too. It is for many of us a time of stress and challenge, but also one of opportunity for maturation and growth.

But, of course, this is not simply about the physical relationship. The one thing you can be sure of when you are having a baby is that life is never going to be the same again. And your relationship with your partnership is never going to be exactly the same again, either.

Most couples are more uneasy about this than they will admit. They concentrate on the birth as if it were a hurdle to be leapt over and feel uncomfortable about discussing the time after the baby comes. I have noticed that their eyes glaze over when the antenatal teacher tries to open a discussion about how a baby affects the partnership. So much is already happening to them during the pregnancy that it may be too much to have to face up to further changes after the birth.

One new father said the baby's arrival was an anti-climax after all this preparation: '*Everything was so fixated on the birth that what followed seemed irrelevant. What were we supposed to do now? I was over-prepared for birth and under-prepared for fatherhood. After the birth we could have gone on quite happily without the baby!*'

Most research on the effects of the baby focuses on things that can go wrong. One of the first sociological studies of parenthood as crisis warned of social isolation, exhaustion, loss of job satisfaction, loss of income, domestic slavery, guilt at being inadequate, an overload of responsibility, financial worries, decline in living standards, loss of libido, depression, and anxiety about getting pregnant again. All this was hammered in further by another study which claimed that babies lead straight to the divorce court.

In many ways our culture programmes couples for disaster. They are told to be ready for marriage breakdown and not about the sense of excitement and self-discovery that comes with coping with stress and meeting challenges. Always thinking in terms of risk and crisis makes it more difficult to deal with problems and prevents adjustment to change. It is like trying to drive with the handbrake on.

That first year after birth is, for many couples, chaos and glory! Your ears strain to hear every sound. You long to sprout additional arms and hands so that you can juggle the baby, clear up the mess, cook a meal and answer the phone.

The woman's entire system, and that of the partner who is fully involved, is geared for emergencies. To care for a baby is to have a new alertness which can be utterly exhausting, especially the first time round. If your baby cries it is as if there were an alarm clock ticking away inside the child, and at the first buzz and whirr you are ready for it. You dread it getting a start on you and ringing and ringing so that you can do nothing about it, cannot turn it off, and are powerless to silence it.

Sam and Rachel's baby's crying time lasted from six to 11pm. That is a common pattern and one that comes as a shock to new parents. Rachel said, *'When Sam comes in he makes me a drink and then holds the baby while I make dinner. Then I hold him while he eats. Then he holds him while I eat. We have never had a meal that wasn't on our laps. Our social life has come to an abrupt stop.'* Though Rachel enjoys getting dressed up and going out, she says it is now out of the question.

Though they talk a lot to each other, it is about different subjects now. *'Conversations about politics, for example, are crowded out, and anything you need time to explore. Now it's simply logistics. We end up talking about the baby 90 per cent of the time.'*

When the same thing happened to Bruce and Wendy they decided to plan for a quiet time together at least once a week. *'Before we had him we used to have a bath together on Saturday afternoons, go to bed and make love, and then get up for dinner out. We miss that. Then my sister said she'd have the baby for two hours. So instead of going out for dinner, we have a take-away when we collect him. That space was just what was needed.'*

But it is not only a question of having no time to be alone. There may be emotional processes which are difficult to understand. For each partner there may be some grieving. The birth of a child, especially the first, is also a kind of death. They need to be able to relinquish an image of themselves as children or adolescents and come to terms with a new image of themselves as parents. Their relationship, however spontaneous before, may seem set like cement, no longer intimate but institutionalised. In fact their own parents may express relief that they have 'settled down'. The individual who is working outside the home considers that work the 'real' work, and it is usually the woman who is left with the baby clinging to her like a limpet on a rock. The mother has surrendered her personal space, the envelope of identity which defined who she was. It is exciting, yet painful, to have that envelope peeled off and know that you are exposed, vulnerable to a baby's need of you. Through the first three or four months after birth – sometimes longer – it is normal for a woman to be tied by an emotional cord to her baby. If such an obsessional concentration on another human being occurred at any other time in our lives it might be diagnosed as a psychiatric illness.

With a first baby, a woman is often striving to do everything perfectly. Being a parent is a highly self-conscious activity. We struggle to mother perfectly in order to produce the ideal baby, who will become a socially well-adjusted toddler who can read and write before he or she is three, and so on through childhood and adolescence. Such goal-orientated parenting imposes its own burdens and means that from the very moment when a woman first takes her baby in her arms, and wants to 'bond' immediately, it is as if she is going in for a series of examinations in motherhood.

The partner may feel shut out from the intimate relationship between the biological mother and baby. Sometimes unresolved early hostility towards a younger brother or sister and the fear of losing the parent's love is sparked off again by the birth of a baby. One who was an only child may never have learned to share a love, even while getting enormous pleasure from seeing the mother and baby together, there may be a twinge of jealousy.

Even when a woman has an intact perineum she may worry that after the birth her vagina will be vast and cavernous. She imagines that if the baby's head is going to be able to get out she will be so stretched that her tissues will hang like sagging washing on a clothes line.

In fact, this rarely happens. The mucus membrane lining of the vagina is flexible and opens up and closes like a concertina. The muscles inside – a circle clasping the vagina about half way up and other deeper layers which support the bladder and uterus – may sag at first, but with pelvic floor movements can be toned in six to eight weeks. A mistake often made is to tackle the pelvic floor only at exercise sessions, where it needs good internal posture all the time and mobilisation of the muscles to get them as expressive as those around the mouth. Good posture comes easily if you think of a smile. Greet each morning with a pelvic floor smile.

If the partner has been with the mother during the birth, sharing and helping, he or she is likely to feel in awe and wonder at her power to produce life. Some men gain a new respect and understanding of the female body. But when birth has been highly medicalised with tubes and gadgets sticking from almost every orifice, he may be frightened and anxious that his sexual feelings can lead to a medical crisis and cause pain. If he has felt needed in labour – when she has sought his eyes as every contraction started, gained strength from his love and has given birth in his arms – there is often a new tenderness and surprising joy at lovemaking after the baby is born.

That first year post-baby is a challenge to a relationship. Even when a partner gives loving support, a mother may feel completely trapped as she tries to meet the baby's needs. It is not only that life is disrupted. The normal divisions of time between day and night are obliterated and she struggles to hold on to a bit of her own space, but it is constantly eroded. If it is the second or third time round, she may also have to cope with a demanding toddler learning to handle feelings of jealousy of the new baby. When it is the first baby and she is accustomed to a job which enables her to complete each task, check and then start another, motherhood comes as a shock because she can never finish anything she is doing.

And yet . . . life is transmuted, emblazoned with excitement, the revelation of a baby's personality. One new mother told me, '*We marvel at the reality of the human being we have both created. We tiptoe in at night and look at him and hug each other with pleasure. His crying is enormously taxing, but he has made us have to cope and that has been good for us and emphasised our partnership.*'

There is new life to discover, a new person to get to know, and an astonishing flood of love flowing through a couple's whole being. You feel more alive than before, more in tune with each other and with the life-force that has swept both of you up into this utterly demanding and deeply satisfying experience.

Sex and Breastfeeding

When you have had your baby you may be longing to get back to 'normal' as soon as possible, or – on the other hand – may enjoy the different way your body feels and looks. Breastfeeding, and your confidence about it, will affect how you think about your body.

However much you enjoy being a mother your new role is bound to be stressful. There are things you have to learn and challenges you need to confront. Your whole way of life changes. The relationship between you and your partner evolves, with your baby now an important part of it. Worrying about not feeling sexually aroused makes this transition more difficult. So take one day at a time. If you had a good relationship before the baby came you will find it again once you relax and the baby becomes integrated into the changing flow of your lives.

Some women are less interested in genital sex when they breastfeed. For them breastfeeding is simply a nurturing task, and a satisfying one – which gives a closeness to the baby that helps them get to know him or her. In the early weeks, and sometimes months, of breastfeeding many women are not sexually aroused in a way they have been before, and do not enjoy genital sex with their partner. If you are facing difficulties in breastfeeding you probably do not feel at all good about your body, but think of it as cumbersome and awkward. This, in turn, affects how you feel about genital sex. If you are trying to cope with breastfeeding problems you are likely to be anxious about them, and have little or no energy or time for erotic sexual feelings.

A woman who has survived sexual abuse may find it particularly hard to relax when she breastfeeds. She may have flashbacks to abuse when a man sucked or bit her breasts. However, for some women who have been abused breastfeeding is empowering, since they are using their bodies in a positive way. And a woman who starts off feeling that the baby is yet another person who is abusing her often starts to enjoy breastfeeding once it is well established.

Other women discover, occasionally to their surprise, that

breastfeeding is an elating experience and brings to their bodies a delicious sensitivity and a feeling of fulfilment. A woman who relishes breastfeeding may feel sexually aroused as her baby tugs and sucks. These feelings make some women feel ashamed and guilty. But it is normal to have intense physical pleasure in breastfeeding, and occasionally even to have an orgasm as a result.

Most of us probably experience both these feelings at different times. We veer between just managing to fit breastfeeds into our busy lives and experiencing them as deeply satisfying, even blissful.

Some Physical Effects of Breastfeeding

While you are breastfeeding you may be aware that your vagina is especially dry, even when sexually aroused. This is because during lactation the level of oestrogen circulating in your blood is lower than usual. If you wish to have intercourse, use a lubricant that either you or your partner strokes into the dry tissues – you can make this a pleasurable part of lovemaking. In the first weeks of breastfeeding your nipples may feel tender and sore and any nipple stimulation in lovemaking hurts. Pressure on your breasts may be painful while you are lactating, too, especially if they are full, because a feed is due shortly. Your partner should avoid putting weight on your breasts or squeezing them during lovemaking. The 'missionary' position for intercourse is usually uncomfortable for this reason, unless he takes his weight on his elbows.

Babies have an uncanny sixth sense that seems to tell them when you are making love. That's the time when they decide they need to be fed. Rather than coitus interruptus, this is 'baby interruptus'. The best time to enjoy leisurely lovemaking is immediately a baby has settled after a feed.

Perhaps you feel that you want to make love but not to have intercourse. Lovemaking after childbirth lets you explore together ways of arousing and satisfying each other that are far more complex and enriching than simple penetration and ejaculation. Some men who have previously ejaculated fast learn to prolong lovemaking so that it is much more satisfying for the woman, and as they slow down they become gentler. A woman may discover she feels intense sexual arousal when her partner is using a little finger or a tenderly searching mouth.

A woman who is breastfeeding may not want her partner, whether male or female, making love to her breasts, even though she enjoyed it before the baby was born, and will again when lactation is over. She may feel that her breasts belong to the baby and it is difficult to mix in her mind the sensations that her baby and her lover arouse. On the other hand, she may welcome her partner's touch and be happy about drawing her lover to her breasts. But a man may feel anxious about touching or sucking her breasts, and carefully avoids any contact with them.[143] The important thing is to be open about how you feel and to recognise that there are no rules about how you should behave.

As you experience orgasm there is a sudden surge of oxytocin, the hormone that stimulates the milk ejection reflex. This pours into your bloodstream and milk may spurt from your breasts. It can feel wonderful. But some women hold back from reaching a climax because they dislike this involuntary milk ejection, or are aware that their partner dislikes it, and think it is messy. The flow of milk during lovemaking is part of your body's richness and vitality in the same way that juices are released around your cervix within your vagina, your whole body becomes hot and damp, and your eyes shine and cheeks glow during intense sexual excitement.

If you have put on a lot of weight in pregnancy it can take some weeks – or months – to lose it again after the birth. So you may be feeling very hefty, and this negative body image puts you off sex. Women who are breastfeeding, on the other hand, lose this weight faster, on average, than bottle-feeding mothers.

It is lovely having the baby sleeping close to or with you both, on the outside of the bed for safety. If this means that you are more tuned into the baby than your lover, buy a cradle that snaps onto the side of the bed or put the baby in a crib at arm's length. For some women having the infant near is so off-putting that they prefer to put the baby in another room for a while – a potent signal to a partner that they would like to make love!

The important thing to realise is that there is a wide range of feelings and that goal-orientated sex – feeling under pressure to have an orgasm – destroys spontaneous pleasure. Others say that breastfeeding makes them more aware of their sexuality and enhances genital sex.[144]

They may worry that she will never be able to enjoy sex again. They have reduced libido, less intercourse and fewer orgasms while breastfeeding,[145] but find that their sex drive returns in full force when the baby is weaned. If she enjoyed genital sex before, she will enjoy it again.

But research results are conflicting, which suggests that both types of reaction, and a range of behaviour in between, are normal. One study showed that three quarters of breastfeeding women do not notice any difference in their sexual feelings after childbirth.[146] A sizable minority, however, said that they were less interested in intercourse while they were breastfeeding. Once they weaned the baby everything was the same as before. Another study revealed that women who breastfeed start intercourse again sooner after the birth than those who do not, report less pain during the postpartum period and also enjoy sex more.[147]

Explanations for a lowered sex drive range from the common sense ('she's tired out; how can you expect her to be sexy?') through the psychoanalytical ('the substitution of the love object') and the hormonal ('prolactin is anti-sex'). A breastfeeding woman's uterus contracts strongly and goes back to its pre-pregnancy size and position earlier than the uterus of one who is bottle-feeding.

Anyone with a baby needing feeds every two or three hours feels that her body belongs to her baby. When her breasts fill up and ache because it is time for the baby to suckle, but she is at a party, she realises just how physically dependent she is on the child. She needs the baby as much as the baby needs her.

It is difficult for couples who were already facing sexual difficulties before the pregnancy started. Having a baby is not going to solve their problems and adds extra stresses which result in further deterioration of the relationship. It may be a good time to seek help from a counsellor.

Some women find breastfeeding exciting and are acutely responsive to breast stimulation.[148] Even those who do not breastfeed may experience heightened breast eroticism. A woman who discovers that she is sexually stimulated by her baby's suckling may feel embarrassed that two separate categories of body experience are getting confused.

A more common difficulty is that a woman gets so used to responding to the baby that she cannot 'switch gears' and respond to her lover's touch.

However sex after birth turns out to be for you, whatever problems you confront, enjoy your baby together. Take this opportunity of a new closeness to explore different ways of making love that give expression to your caring and tenderness for each other.

12

CHANGING CHILDBIRTH

Three huge changes occurred in childbirth over the last half-century. In the USA medicalisation of birth was already well under way by the 1960s. Women were routinely strapped, wrists and ankles tied, flat on their backs, drugged into a state of 'twilight sleep', sliced open from the vagina toward the anus, and delivered by forceps. New interventions were proposed intended to make birth easier. Many of them led to more procedures that made birth more and more complicated and frightening.

Some highly eccentric technological inventions, intended to make birth easier for women and babies, were never introduced. Take the 'Blonsky' for example. Jennifer Block, an investigative journalist, opens her vividly written book *Pushed* by describing 'apparatus for facilitating the birth of a child by centrifugal force'.[149] The idea was that instead of being manacled, drugged, cut and having a forceps delivery, the mother would be strapped to a hefty machine that generated power up to seven times the force of gravity. George and Lotta Blonsky, who never had children themselves but were shocked by what women had to go through in US hospitals, were fascinated by seeing an elephant at the zoo giving birth. They claimed that she whirled round in circles. Their preposterous invention was intended to imitate this movement by whirling the mother around at high speed.

The expulsive power produced would have been greater than that experienced by astronauts taking off into space. The mother would certainly have blacked out. Astronauts wear special clothing to counteract the force of three Gs at lift-off. This contraption would have generated seven Gs. And no-one knows what would have happened to the baby.

Whatever the Blonskys witnessed in the zoo, it was odd. An elephant giving birth in the wild is normally surrounded by other female elephants, and does not spin in circles. It sounds as if a panic-stricken animal was struggling to escape from a cage.

Styles of medical and surgical management that start in the USA give a picture of what will happen elsewhere some years later.

In the UK a major change was a move from home to hospital. But about a third of mothers still had their babies at home 50 years ago. Today only three in 100 do so.

When birth was taken outside the home and subjected to institutional management women became treated as containers to be opened and relieved of their contents within strictly limited time constraints, and attention was concentrated on a bag of muscle and a birth canal, rather than a person.

Along with this change in the place of birth came a change in the person making decisions about the conduct of labour. It was no longer the midwife. There was a take-over by obstetricians, though their main interest was not normal birth but gynaecology. A doctor's status in the medical system derived from that. The midwife did most of the work, but was a subservient member of a team, assisting its senior members, and obeying protocols set by the institution. The result was a loss of satisfaction in her work, and, because they had to obey institutional protocols, for the majority of those in large hospitals an inestimable reduction in personal caring, skilled observation, and understanding of the woman in childbirth. Midwives lost out and mothers lost out, together.

The third overwhelming change, and part and parcel of it, was the technology revolution. Investigations and intervention started early in pregnancy.

Delivery rooms came to resemble torture chambers, and in the words of one obstetrician – not a radical one – 'Labour wards looked like some scientific hell hole, with instruments everywhere and flashing lights'.

Clinical skills were lost and replaced by technology, a

technology which would be intrusive under any conditions, but in practice was still more disturbing because it often went wrong, and because hospital staff often did not know how to interpret the data spewing out of the machinery.

Electronic fetal monitoring during labour is a case in point. It replaced intermittent auscultation of the baby's heart and leads to more unnecessary interventions, without evidence that it saves babies' lives or reduces cerebral palsy.[150]

It meant that women could no longer trust their bodies. In fact, their bodies had become enemies. This is still how it is in many hospitals. Spontaneous feelings are rejected, as women in labour are required to put on a performance in an alien environment, often in front of total strangers. For those who have been through that ordeal references to the sexuality of birth must sound like the ravings of someone who is severely mentally disturbed.

'The history of Western obstetrics is the history of technologies of separation. We've separated milk from breasts, mothers from babies, fetuses from pregnancies, sexuality from procreation, pregnancy from motherhood. And finally we're left with the image of the fetus as a free-floating being alone, analogous to man in space, with the umbilical cord tethering the placental ship, and the mother reduced to the empty space that surrounds it.'[151]

The obstetric view of childbirth is that it is a medical event conducted by a team of professionals, in an intensive care setting. Pregnancy is a potentially pathological condition, to be terminated by delivery.

A woman who had her first baby in the 1980s described the ordeal of the obstacle race that pregnancy had become, with a general atmosphere of gloom and incipient catastrophe hanging over it. Test followed test, increasing her anxiety as she approached her due date, and she remarked that doctors and midwives are 'forever worrying about dates, and whether the baby is growing at the right speed'. With ultrasound and electronic fetal monitoring women were then – and often still are – subjected to trial by antenatal clinic.

It is taken for granted that antenatal care must be a good thing, but there is little evidence to show that any particular aspects of that care are of value except in the broadest statistical terms. We have only the vaguest idea of *which* women benefit from care, how *much* they need, or exactly what *kind* of care. Antenatal care may damage a woman's perception of her body and her feeling that she can work with it. It is then counter-productive.

Risk Management

Risk is often over-estimated in pregnancy and this affects everything that is done to women and how they feel about their bodies. 'Ultimately obstetric care is complex and efforts to avoid pre-natal risk exposure based on heightened perceptions of threat may do more harm than the perceived threat itself.'[152] Moreover, 'When people have been given a disease label, they often find themselves on a rollercoaster of further tests, associated anxieties and sometimes unjustified discrimination, for example by insurance companies.'[153]

To live under the threat of risk, and being determined to avoid it at all costs, is to be exposed to extreme stress. That eventually could erode our capacity to make any decisions at all. The struggle to avoid risk drains any joyful sexuality from the birth experience. And it exposes us to a host of technocratic interventions, while at the same time minimising the harm that medical procedures can bring.[154]

Concentrating on risk statistics produced as the result of randomised controlled trials published in medical journals renders us unable to see the hidden risks that come from mutilating the birth experience and disrupting the hormonal flow of sexual energy.[155,156]

Dr Marion Hall's work in Aberdeen showed that the productivity of routine antenatal care in prediction and detection of obstetric problems was extremely low, and incorrect diagnosis was common. For every case of intrauterine growth retardation correctly predicted there were 2.5 false positives and for every case of pre-eclampsia or hypertension diagnosed there were another 1.3 false positives. She pointed out that this incorrect diagnosis led to extensive investigation and unnecessary admission to hospital for induction resulting in some cases in forceps delivery and Caesarean section.[157] Antenatal procedures are ritualised in order to institutionalise the passage through pregnancy and the behaviour of every woman who passes through it. In the process a woman is de-sexed.

In 1981 I initiated and chaired a working party on antenatal care for the National Childbirth Trust. We were mothers, fathers, midwives, obstetricians, hospital administrators and other health professionals. In our report we stated that:

'The average hospital antenatal clinic is a major problem area within the National Health Service. From all over Britain women's accounts of their experiences of care indicate that: The expectant mother is treated as the passive object of management, who is fed into the system and whose progress through it from point to point is controlled as if she had no wishes or preferences of her own.

Clinics are often a long way from where those they are intended to service actually live or work. (And even if a clinic is eight miles away having to go on two different buses with a toddler and a push-chair makes it an arduous journey.)

Waiting times are long, often two hours or more, and sometimes exceed three hours, in surroundings that are often extremely uncomfortable and frequently depressing. Few hospitals provide anything for women to do except wait. Facilities for child care are usually absent and playthings rarely provided. Toddlers become fractious and weary. Clinics are often grossly overcrowded and have the atmosphere of a badly managed cattlemarket.

There is an almost complete absence of continuity of care and each time she attends a woman sees different, anonymous faces and may also be given conflicting information and advice, which leads to anxiety and confusion.

Contact with the obstetrician is restricted to one or two minutes. To many women this seems the whole point of the visit, and all the planning and waiting are directed towards this moment. But for most the visit culminates in only a brief laying on of hands by a member of the obstetric team who may have no more idea of who the person is he is examining than she does of him. It is not surprising that women feel disappointed when they are in and out of the examination room in a matter of minutes and have no opportunity for discussion or for voicing anxieties.

Doctors are not always available in antenatal clinics and block-booked women sit waiting for their appearance. The assumption is that though a doctor should never have to wait for a woman it is acceptable for women to have to wait to see doctors and that the doctor's time is more valuable than the patient's.

Women who are most at risk, who include a large proportion of those from deprived socio-economic backgrounds, are those least likely to get the care they need.'[158]

To turn the process of bringing new life into the world into one in which a woman is a passive patient being delivered, rather than an active birth-giver responding to the signals coming from her body in a spontaneous way, is to degrade her. Nor is the right to 'control' her body in childbirth to do with dominating it, as Russian and French psychoprophylaxis taught. Rather, it means trusting it to tell her what to do, and when and how.

Films on TV depict the second stage as the culmination of a desperate race in which a woman is bullied to force a large object through a very small hole. But the urge to push is involuntary. Although sometimes compared to a sneeze, it is much more like mounting to orgasm, in wave after wave of desire. Pain can seem irrelevant compared with the urgency of longing and the triumphant, glorious opening of the vagina through which the baby slides.

Witch-hunts

In Britain Wendy Savage, consultant obstetrician in Tower Hamlets, who worked closely with GP obstetricians, attended home births, ran courses for GPs called 'Home Birth for the

Hesitant' and supported vaginal birth after previous Caesarean section when women wanted it, was suspended from practice in 1985, following long-standing disagreements with male hospital colleagues, who banded together to oust her.[159]

Her suspension was a direct attack on the concept of community obstetrics. She provided consultant cover for the GPs and there was evidence that it improved continuity and women were more satisfied with this care. Tower Hamlets has a large immigrant population and many women don't want to be attended by a male obstetrician.

Iain Chalmers, then Director of the National Epidemiology Unit in Oxford, wrote in the *Lancet*: 'It goes without saying that inferences about the relative merits and demerits of particular policies should not be based on individual cases selected to make a point but on representative and sufficiently large samples managed by the consultants being compared.'

Women rose up in protest against Wendy Savage's suspension. The Association for Improvements in Maternity Services organised a highly publicised and successful march to support her, and some 5,000 people, predominantly women, came out on the streets. The subsequent enquiry exonerated her completely. It is significant that two months after she was suspended she was awarded a Fellowship of the Royal College of Obstetricians and Gynaecologists.

Questions raised by this witch-hunt are:

1. Is birth exclusively a matter of medical expertise or to do with a woman's body, and her feelings, beliefs and relationships?
2. Is birth to be controlled by medicine or the woman?
3. Are interventions evaluated by rigorous controlled research or part of 'just in case obstetrics'?

If we were forced to make love in public, and in the setting of the standard hospital delivery room, we would probably feel inhibited. If at the same time there were professionals who examined us intra-vaginally, insisted on eye contact, and constrained and cajoled us about what we should do, exactly when, and urged us to speed up and 'try harder', it would be difficult to relax, to centre down into our sensations, and allow a spontaneous flow of hormones in the bloodstream. It would be almost impossible to reach orgasm. Yet this is still the environment most women face in childbirth.

Witch-hunt in Hungary

In the countries of Eastern Europe regimentation of birth derived from Communism is combined with authoritarian obstetrics typical of US maternity care to produce a strict management of childbirth which deprives women of information, allows them no choice, and disempowers them.[160]

In Hungary in September 2007 Ágnes Geréb, an obstetrician who had been struck off for attending home births, who then trained as a midwife, attended a home birth that was entirely straightforward until the moment of delivery. Labour started spontaneously four days after the estimated delivery date, the baby was in an excellent position and of average size, and the liquor was clear. The fetal heart rate gave no cause for concern either in the first or the second stage. The head was born, with a good colour, and the cord was not around the neck. But then the shoulders got stuck. Agnes tried every manoeuvre to correct shoulder dystocia, including the Gaskin manoeuvre (half kneeling-half squatting), but did not perform an episiotomy or fracture the mother's symphysis pubis. An ambulance was called to transport her to the hospital two minutes away, where obstetricians worked to deliver the infant. Sadly, the baby showed no signs of life and could not be resuscitated. It was the first time that this had occurred with a home birth in Hungary.

An inquiry took place and the distressed parents sued Agnes. There was widespread publicity and the media hounded her. She could not go into a store without being stared at. She was found guilty of malpractice, largely because she had not done an episiotomy, and sentenced to house arrest.

Reporters lingered by her front door, and there have been endless abusive anonymous phone calls. She is guilty of a crime the punishment for which is imprisonment. As I write the court has confirmed the guilty verdict and doubled the sentence from five to ten years.

Home birth is now illegal in Hungary, or at least, home birth that is not attended by an obstetrician and a neonatologist with at least ten years' experience. An unlikely situation!

Choice

Through the 1990s much of the debate between women in the birth movement and health professionals concerned 'freedom to choose'. In the USA the American College of Nurse-Midwives, the Midwives Alliance of North America, and the National Association of Parents and Professionals for Safe Alternatives in Childbirth, in response to WHO's call for minimal intervention in childbirth, said 'Our concern is that most women do not currently have access to a model of care that supports normal, physiologic birth' and consequently they have limited options. When women 'choose' medical interventions, it may be with insufficient information, as well as inadequate access to care options that can minimise these interventions.

Birth Plans

One way a pregnant woman can make it more likely that she has a birth environment in which she feels secure and relaxed is to think through her priorities and make a birth plan. She then talks it through with her midwife and whoever is going to be her birth companion.

But for many women who are programmed into the hospital system it is impossible to do this because when labour starts they confront nameless strangers.

After a close colleague of mine in Seattle, Penny Simkin, introduced birth plans into the USA in 1980 I did the same in the UK.[161,162]

Already by 1987 one in every three English hospitals stated that they encouraged women to make birth plans.

The booking clinic (the first hospital antenatal clinic a pregnant woman attends) provides an opportunity to start out on this. At some hospitals a midwife asks as a matter of course, 'Have you thought ahead to the kind of birth you'd like to have? How would you like to deal with labour pain?' and 'Who do you want with you?' Some hospitals provide booklets in which a woman can keep a diary of pregnancy, writing anything she wants to discuss with the midwife or doctor, and record her wishes. There may also be reminders about questions she has on subjects such as labour ward procedures, drugs for pain relief, or what life is like on a postnatal ward – and the choices open to her.

Birth plans are a big issue in childbirth – whether or not to make them, whether they do more harm than good, and exactly how a woman should compile one to get the birth experience she wants.

At present a midwife meets each woman attending the booking clinic for the first time and takes her history. This should be a chance for her to get to know her as a person and help her think about birth plans. But that phrase 'taking the history' is significant. In many hospitals the woman feels that something important has been 'taken' from her: Her own story of what has happened in the past and her hopes and fears for the future are turned into items on a form written in officialese. It is like seeing your statement to the police translated into police language and becoming something you cannot recognise as yourself. Not only may a woman's words be turned into gobbledegook in an antenatal history – whether or not she smokes and the social support she has during pregnancy and after the baby is born – but a host of important issues may not be recorded.

A study of antenatal history-taking by Dr Lesley Mutch and Dr Rupert Fawdry in the *Journal of Obstetrics and Gynaecology* revealed that even in teaching hospitals (and these are probably the best) only half the completed histories contained any information about whether the pregnant woman wanted to breast or bottle-feed her baby. Only four out of 41 hospitals left any space on the form for a woman's feelings about epidurals, and none at all asked her views about different birth positions.[163]

Women are invited to make choices between alternatives. But choices are illusory unless we have information about the consequences of making that choice, the short and long-term side-effects, if any, and the alternatives available. Questions to ask should include, 'Who did the research? Was it in their self-interest to reach a particular conclusion? What methods of enquiry were used? Was it a randomised controlled trial? Was it one-dimensional or did it take into account the total physiological, emotional and social outcomes?' It is vital to incorporate women's experiences of interventions in birth. Yet often the approach is basically 'tick the boxes'.

An advertisement states, 'Eight out of ten women said that *Youth Serum* reduced the visible effects of wrinkles in ten days.' That's one kind of research. Is it convincing? Surprisingly, for many magazine readers, yes. They go off and buy the product.

Birth interventions and invasive technology may be sold in a similar way and are verified by women themselves who give them personal endorsement and are thankful that they had the intervention, or were in hospital, because the baby needed resuscitating, or they were on the spot for a Caesarean. Dilatation was slow, so labour was speeded up with artificial hormones, and they could have an epidural. Women who have had a previous traumatic birth, and those who have suffered sexual abuse which may dominate their thinking about birth, want to escape pain and have expectations that certain techniques will make birth painless. The effects of the environment itself and on relationships with caregivers are often ignored, and the overwhelming impact of fear on mind and body.

Doctors and midwives sometimes regard the woman who produces a birth plan as a potential troublemaker, and occasionally become hostile because of this perceived threat to their professional skills. Even those keen to make birth a satisfying experience may tense up and become suspicious because, they tell me, 'Birth plans shouldn't be necessary. What is important is the relationship of trust.' That can't, in one doctor's words, 'be mandated by contract'. He went on to explain that some women presented pages of requests and that he always felt bad about these for three reasons.

First, they had presupposed that he was not prepared to give them what they wanted unless they wrote it down. Secondly, it was often those women with the most precise plans who experienced the kind of birth that they didn't anticipate, and thirdly, as a result, both he and the woman felt afterwards that they had failed.

There is no doubt that the laundry list approach to birth plans causes problems. A woman – especially if it is her first pregnancy – cannot know how she will feel or exactly what she will want when in labour. She may have hoped for a group of friends with her, but when it comes to it all she longs for is peace and quiet and one trusted supporter, or even to be left alone. She may be determined to have no painkillers, but undergo a long and difficult labour and decide to have an epidural. Producing a rigid list of requests means that she cannot be flexible and that she and her caregivers feel bound by a set of rules.

Every birth is a journey of discovery and it is vitally important for the woman *and* her helpers to be adaptable and open to new ideas. Making a birth plan can be an opportunity for collaboration between them. It should be a *process* rather than an act, a shared learning experience rather than the issuing of a manifesto.

But it isn't only pregnant women who may not understand how to use a birth plan. It is not that women don't know *how* to use it, but they may have greater expectations of it than are realistic. A major problem is that many midwives and doctors do not comprehend the whole birth plan idea and are ignorant of how it can enable them to get on the same wavelength as the woman whom they should be serving. In some hospitals which use birth plans women are asked to fill in forms, ticking 'Yes/No' boxes in response to questions about whether they want to wear a hospital gown or their own nightie, have the lights dimmed for delivery or not, hold the baby or not, and so on. This not only trivialises the concept of birth plans but, because it introduces the idea of choice while at the same time framing and restricting possible alternatives, it gives women the impression that they have choices when they have none.

It is all very well being presented with a selection of set menus, but suppose what you want is not on the menu at all? A woman who dares to ask for something that has not been offered – and that can take a lot of courage – feels like a shopper who is told 'There is no demand for it, Madam', and so she must be a freak.

Such a system marginalises anyone wanting something that is not already done in the hospital. One result is that medical practices become enshrined and do not change.

In every country when formal birth plans are introduced by hospitals they risk being just a sop to quieten consumer demands. It is as if the hospital is saying, 'Look how progressive we are. You can have your baby any way you like here, within reason.' Many women who have already had babies have learned to be very suspicious of obstetricians who say, 'You can have your baby hanging from the chandeliers as far as I'm concerned' and '*Of course* you can give birth naturally. *All* birth is natural!' They invariably discover that these obstetricians are autocratic, paternalistic and rigid in their management of labour – even if they are women. The same healthy distrust should be brought to hospital-compiled birth plans.

It is this nervous mothering of child-bearing women on the part of some midwives which dismisses birth plans on the grounds that they make patients 'unnecessarily anxious'. The idea is that the less information women have, the better. They can relax only if they hand over decisions to professionals, knowing that they are in safe hands. To support this argument some doctor friends – men every one of them – have told me that they wouldn't want to know the details of any surgical operation they were about to have, or make choices about the care they were given after a coronary.

There are flaws in this argument. First, no-one suggests that women should be *forced* to make decisions. Second, a woman having a baby is usually not ill. She may be at the peak of health. She often wants to know what is going on, to make informed choices between alternatives, and share in all decisions made about her body and her baby.

Yet those doctors and midwives who say that birth plans

shouldn't be necessary have a case. For it is true that if the doctor or midwife understands what is in the woman's mind, and wants to help her give birth in whatever way she wishes, plans could be superfluous. The two are in partnership and do not need their dialogue formalised.

But the vast majority of women do not have a one-to-one relationship with those who are looking after them. In hospitals continuity of care is not only difficult to guarantee, but almost impossible to achieve. No woman wants the way she is treated in labour to depend on whoever happens to be on duty at the moment. The birth plan process is a way of creating a dialogue and recording its cumulative outcome, so that any member of staff can refer to it and understand the woman's wishes. It is often the only means of providing continuity when there are constantly changing personnel, care is task-orientated and women give birth in an alien environment among strangers. Those are the conditions under which most babies are born in technocratic cultures today.

Chopping Off the End of Pregnancy

Labours are induced and elective Caesareans performed to cut pregnancy short in the belief that babies are safer out once there are only a few more weeks of pregnancy to go, and that mothers – and incidentally obstetricians – want to plan ahead. Labour often takes hours, sometimes days. So scheduling surgery seems to be an efficient, cost-effective way of managing birth that is otherwise unpredictable.

There are other reasons too: a growing epidemic of obesity, for example. But they are trivial beside the obstetric interventions that dictate the date and time of birth.

Pregnancy is estimated to last 40 weeks. Perhaps 39 weeks doesn't sound all that different. But there are risks. Between 1992 and 2002 the percentage of full-term births in the United States declined by more than 20%, while 'late preterm births' (between 34 and 36 weeks) went up by 12 per cent. They have a greater likelihood of breathing problems, feeding difficulties, temperature instability (hypothermia), jaundice and reduced brain development than full-term babies.'[164] Mothers of late preterm babies are more likely to confront breastfeeding problems because these babies are not quite ready neurologically for the major adaptations to life outside the uterus.

Obstetricians are often unaware that these babies have problems. Dr David Savitz, an epidemiologist at Mount Sinai Medical Center, New York, who studies trends in preterm birth says, 'When you look at large populations, there are small but very real increases in the risk of adverse outcomes for those 34, 35 or 36 week babies, but it may be something that an individual clinician never sees.'

Occasionally, in spite of ultrasound (which can give a date two weeks out either way), the experts get it wrong and a baby who is thought to be 36 or 38 weeks turns out to be 32 or 34 weeks, and needs to be sent to the intensive care nursery for help with breathing and nasogastric feeding.

A baby can plump up by half a pound a week at the end of pregnancy, and this additional growth prepares it for the challenges of life. That extra time being rocked in the cradle of the mother's pelvis as she moves, hearing the steady drumming of her heartbeat, and being nourished directly from her bloodstream as it is filtered through the placenta helps the baby mature.

Even if the baby is ready to be born, induction changes the physiology of birth. When labour is kick-started the mother may need strong painkilling drugs because huge contractions come in quick succession and she feels helpless, as if drowning in a storm at sea. So she has an epidural. Then the baby's heart rate drops and drugs are used to stimulate it. After birth both mother and baby may develop a fever – a common side-effect of epidurals – so they have to go through a series of tests for infection.

An epidural makes labour longer, especially at the pushing stage. When a mother has no spontaneous desire to push she finds it difficult to work with her body to get the baby out and, because the epidural causes loss of tone in her pelvic floor muscles, the baby's head may not rotate to get in the best position for birth. All this increases the chance of an instrumental delivery using forceps or vacuum extraction, or an emergency Caesarean section. A high proportion of planned early deliveries are either elective Caesareans or failed inductions that end up as emergency sections.

Induction of labour and the Caesarean section that often results leaves many women distressed in the months after birth. At first they feel relieved that they have got through the ordeal and the baby has come. Then, after some weeks or months, it hits them. They were denied any control over the way the baby came into the world and were just a body on the delivery table. Some feel violated. But they are supposed to be grateful to the medical system that did this to them. People tell them they should be happy they have a healthy baby, and urge them to put it behind them and get on with their lives. Intense memories of the birth go round and round in their heads like a video tape that cannot be switched off. They suffer nightmares, flashbacks and panic attacks. This is post-traumatic stress disorder. Their unhappiness affects how they feel about the baby, about themselves as women, and their partners.[165]

Childbirth is not only a matter of having a live baby and a live mother. The way it is conducted, the setting where it takes place, and every intervention, even if routine, needs to be evaluated in terms of the physical and emotional outcomes, for the baby and the mother.

The technocractic management of pregnancy teaches women that their bodies threaten their babies' survival. They may be told that the baby is 'better out than in', and labour is induced or a preterm Caesarean is performed. Rather than finding pleasure in their nurturing bodies, they see them as prisons from which obstetricians enable their babies to escape.

Opting for A Planned Caesarean

Some women who have been traumatised by childbirth – either one that was an agonising vaginal birth or an emergency Caesarean – see a planned Caesarean as a way to evade the ordeal with another baby. For some this may be the answer. For others it is no solution and will bring more physical and psychological trauma.

A Caesarean is major surgery with both short and long-term side-effects. Post-operative pain may be severe, a baby may have breathing problems at birth and need resuscitation, so may be sent to the intensive care nursery. The painkilling drugs the mother receives are absorbed in breastmilk and passed to the baby. It is more difficult to establish breastfeeding after a Caesar so extra patience is needed. A Caesarean also introduces the risk of placenta praevia, an adherent placenta and rupture of the scar. Only non-randomised studies have been published, but vaginal birth is an option and if uterine stimulants are avoided research suggests that when there has been a smaller lower segment incision for a Caesarean – which is usually the case nowadays – it makes another pregnancy nothing like as risky as it used to be when women were still sliced open right down the uterus.

So a woman who missed the hormonal rhythms of labour in a previous birth may still be able, if she is in a stress-free environment and with sensitive, non-intrusive support, to relish the hormonal rhythms of labour and have a vaginal birth with her next baby.

Planned Caesareans for Breech Birth

'*My baby was breech and although I really wanted to have a normal birth, the consultant waved his hand in the air and said, "Do you want your baby to die?" and gave me a date to come in for a cesarean. I was too frightened to refuse.*'[166]

A Canadian randomised controlled trial published in 2000[167,168] had a dramatic effect on the management of breech births. Vaginal delivery was dismissed as too dangerous; it caused death and morbidity in babies. From then on breech presentation dictated Caesarean delivery.

Yet when the vaginal births in this randomised controlled study were examined closely it was clear that there were a host of confounding variables. Many of the vaginal breech births were managed intrusively and aggressively, following induction, augmentation and physical manipulation. These vaginal births were not studied in depth.

Kathleen Fahy[169] examined a list of protocols for the aggressive management of breech births assembled by Maggie Banks.[170] It looks as if this busy and intrusive management could have been harmful. It included induction and augmentation of labour, auscultation of the fetal heart every 15 minutes or continuous ECG, the mother heavily drugged and passive and not allowed anything to eat or drink through labour, pulling down the baby's body or legs when the body was born to the umbilicus, and delivery of the head either with forceps or using the Mauriceau-Smellie-Veit manoeuvre.

In contrast, midwives experienced with spontaneous vaginal breech births helped create a warm, safe environment for a woman they already knew, and waited until labour started naturally. They gave no drugs, let her eat and drink during labour, encouraged her to move and change position if she wished, helped her to an upright or semi-upright position for birth, and, with a policy of 'hands off the breech', watched and waited as the body was born spontaneously, using no traction, however gentle, simply supporting the baby's weight while encouraging the mother to listen to her body and do whatever she wanted.

A mother with a breech baby writes:

'Finally I find myself in the delivery suite with the lovely and very experienced midwife. She told me that I was six cm dilated and asked me what I wanted to do. I asked to use the pool and she immediately went and filled it for me. Then she just sat and watched as my body took over as I gave in to my contractions. Only once she sensed a change in the noises I was making did she ask if I felt like pushing and helped me out of the pool and back to my room to birth my baby. I birthed my baby completely unassisted while this wonderful midwife and her supervisor who had come in to oversee the birth just watched and encouraged me. No-one touched me or my baby and there was certainly no talk of stirrups or forceps. I was left to listen to my body and let it take charge of birthing my baby and it rose to the challenge magnificently.'[171]

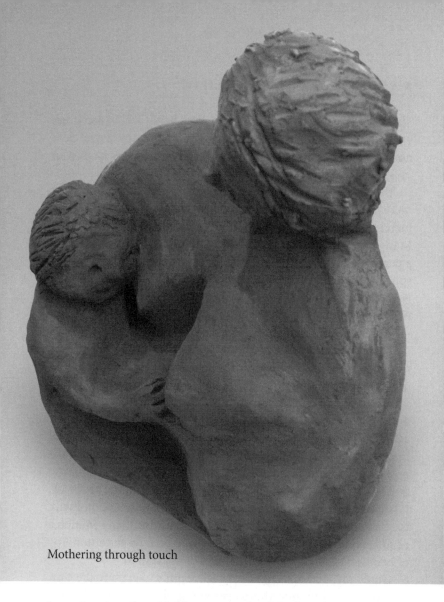

Mothering through touch

Lumping together highly managed vaginal with spontaneous breech births, and comparing all these with Caesarean outcomes, confounds a range of variables, so the study comes to very unreliable conclusions.

This is another way in which women's bodies are treated as containers to be emptied of their contents, another way in which women are denied a psychosexual experience.

Am I Good Enough to be a Mother?

There is increasing emphasis on midwives being able to recognise symptoms of failure in bonding – to detect the woman who does not hold out her arms for her baby, who turns away from it or says it is ugly.

This is one among other very disturbing aspects of our increasing ability to detect when things have gone wrong but our inability to prepare the right soil in which things can go right. Many women who later fall in love with their babies pass through a period following birth when they draw away from the child, in spite of what they want or hoped for. That is not surprising when we consider what is done to their bodies. A woman may need time after birth – to find, to reclaim her body again, to be herself – before she can reach out to her baby.

There is danger that we neglect the nurturing which allows her time to bond with her baby, and force her to pass a first examination in her 'right to be a mother' during the prescribed 'bonding time'.

A vital part of finding yourself again, and getting back into your body and your life, is the chance to be private. When the tubes, catheters and electronics are removed there is a precious interval between the routines of the delivery suite and the routines of the post-partum ward when at last there can be implicit recognition that birth is an intimate, personal experience, and that above all, it belongs to the woman. She needs time, not only to bond with the baby but to make a pattern out of what is for many women a chaotic and fragmented experience – to rediscover the autonomy of being an adult, not a child trapped in the system.

Gradually, perhaps tentatively, she begins to explore the tiny, firm body, to look into those eyes seeing the world for the first time. It is not only that she comes into a relationship with her baby and feels it is hers. In the signals coming from the newborn, who is from the very beginning a social being, the woman is herself acknowledged. It is remarkable how many women, in describing these first 'conversations' with the baby say that the child looked at them as if to say, 'So – that's who my mother is' and comment: 'The baby seemed to know me' or 'I think he recognises my voice'. The mother may say to the baby, 'Hello – yes, it's me!' In this way the woman is validated in her role as the mother by the baby. It is not only that the mother nurtures her baby, but the baby nurtures the woman as a mother.

A very important aspect of this is that the couple who have been together through the experience of birth should be undisturbed as long as they want after the birth. The partner should be able to be in the hospital overnight, and the staff should knock on the door instead of just barging in. What is taking place is not only a bonding of mother and baby, but also of the other parent and baby, and with this a bonding between the two parents.

We need to acknowledge that birth is not the termination of a nine-month disease called pregnancy, but is a psychosexual experience of profound significance. There is growing awareness that the setting for birth has a powerful effect on the way our bodies function, and that a high-tech environment turns it from a psychosexual process into a series of medical/surgical acts.

Today there is lively discourse between women, midwives and other caregivers about the conduct of birth and the environment in which it takes place. Women are increasingly critical of interventionist obstetrics that masquerade as science. Mothers and midwives have come to see that when a woman has freedom to follow her instincts, and allow the creative force to surge through her, birth-giving can be an act of assent to life, a thanksgiving, and in spite of pain, a sexually intense experience. She rides on co-ordinated waves of endocrines released in her bloodstream that stimulate involuntary responses of incredible urgency which open her body, embrace the baby, and press it down to birth.

We are on the threshold of reclaiming spontaneous childbirth.

ACKNOWLEDGEMENTS

This book would never have seen the light of day without help, support and opposition from a wide range of people, many of whom are close friends. I acknowledge that my thinking is stimulated by being challenged, and I am very glad that this is so. Thank you to Janet Balaskas, founder of the Active Birth Movement, for her ideas about moving, rather than static positions, in childbirth, and suggestions for practising these ahead, illustrated on pages 105–110. The brilliant photographs of belly dancing in labour on page 111 are from Maha Al Masa, a birth educator who has brought movements from Arab culture to Australia. Ethel Burns' research into immersion in water has taught me a lot, and her innovative Zumba bumps are illustrated on page 102.

My daughter Nell has created a range of sculptures of childbirth, four of which we included on pages 56, 63, 86 and 175.

Professor Celia Kitzinger introduced me to conversation analysis. Professor Jenny Kitzinger taught me about focus groups, and has always been there to give lively encouragement.

Tess McKenney, another daughter, has taken charge of my computer, given strong back-up and organised study days.

Uwe Kitzinger, my husband, has patiently accepted my working on this book, when he really wanted me to go on holiday with him.

Sue Allen, my assistant, has worked hard and given me strong support, questioning my style of writing and statements in a helpful way.

Dr Michel Odent has explored extensively endocrine elements of spontaneous birth. Dr Murray Enkin built my confidence in what I was trying to do and his humane approach to birth has suffused my work over the years. Other strong influences are

Dr Marsden Wagner, former Director of Child Health for the World Health Organisation in Europe, Sir Iain Chalmers, of the James Lind Alliance, and Professor Nick Fisk in Brisbane, who have supported and encouraged me, and Professor Lesley Page, President of the Royal College of Midwives, who has exceptional insight into sensitive midwifery and is always ready to explore ideas.

Colleagues in the National Childbirth Trust have enabled me to define my views more clearly.

All the women facing birth trauma who have rung me to discuss their experiences have deepened my understanding of what happens when birth is like rape, and the long-term effects of such violence.

The late Betty Parsons, antenatal teacher to royalty, challenged my ideas and was quoted in the press. This led to a furious response from twitterers who claimed that I was mad, instructed me to 'Push it up my fundament', and made other vigorous proposals that are too obscene to quote. It was this that stimulated me to write the book. I want to thank them for insulting me in this way, which drove me to produce *Birth & Sex*.

* * *

I often look at what I'm writing and think, 'I've said that before!' Then I track down where and see that, though I'm changing the focus in this book, it offers useful material that I can't neglect. So *Woman's Experience of Sex* that was published by Dorling Kindersley/Penguin in 1983 provided a mine of material, together with articles I have written for midwifery and childbirth journals and the NCT. Many years of writing, lecturing and research have produced a treasure trove.

REFERENCES

Introduction: Why I write about birth and sex

1   Betty Parsons. Obituary. *The Telegraph*, 6 February 2012. Available from: www.telegraph.co.uk/news/obituaries/9065039/Betty-Parsons.html.

2   Dick-Read G. *Childbirth Without Fear*. London: Harper Collins, 1944.

3   Karmel M. *Thank you, Dr Lamaze*. London: Harper Collins, 1981.

4   Kitzinger S. *The New Experience of Childbirth*. London: Orion, 2004.

5   Kitzinger S. *The Good Birth Guide*. London: Croom Helm, 1979.

6   Kitzinger S. *The New Good Birth Guide*. London: Penguin, 1983.

7   Gaskin IM. *Birth Matters*. London: Pinter and Martin, 2011:52.

Chapter 1: De-sexing birth

8   Groskop V. Yes! Yes! Yes! It's Coming! *The Guardian*, 18 March 2009. Available from: www.guardian.co.uk/lifeandstyle/2009/mar/18/orgasmic-birth-climax-labour.

9   Davis E. *Women, Sex and Desire*. Alameda, CA: Hunter House Publishers, 1995;77.

10 Keverne EB, Levy F, Poindron P, Lindsay DR. Vaginal stimulation: an important determination of maternal bonding in sheep. *Science* 1983;219(4580):81-83.

11 Krehbiel D, Poindron P, Lévy F, Prudhomme MJ. Peridural anesthesia disturbs maternal behavior in primiparous and multiparous parturient ewes. *Physiology and Behavior* 1987;40(4):463-72.

12 Katz Rothman B. *Giving Birth: Alternatives in Childbirth*. Harmondsworth: Penguin, 1982.

13 Katz Rothman B quoted in: Davis-Floyd R, Arvidson PS (eds). *Intuition: The Inside Story*. London: Routledge, 1997;146.

14 Wertz R, Wertz D. *Lying in: A History of Childbirth in America*, London: Free Press, 1977.

15 Consent to treatment. Medical Defence Union, 1974.

16 The Frequency of Unreported Orgasms in Labor and Birth in a Population of Unmedicated Women. 26th Triennial ICM Congress, Vienna, 2002.

17 Patterson I. Orgasm and childbirth. *Times Magazine*, 22 March 2009;37-39.

Chapter 2: Genital geography

18 Hite S. *The Hite Report on Male Sexuality*. London: MacDonald, 1981.

Chapter 3: Sex and pregnancy

19 Cavanagh J, Kelly AJ, Thomas J. Breast stimulation for cervical ripening and induction of labour. *Cochrane Database of Systematic Reviews* 2001;(4):CD003392. Available from: www.cochrane.org.

20 Davis E. *Women, Sex and Desire*. Alameda, CA: Hunter House, 1995;63.

21 Davis E. *op cit.*

Chapter 4: Active birth-giving

22 Masters WH, Johnson VE. *Human Sexual Response*. Boston: Little Brown and Co, 1966.

23 Gersh ES, Gersh I. *The Biology of Women*. London: Junction Books, 1981.

24 Odent M. Fetus ejection reflex and the art of midwifery. Available from: www.wombecology.com/?pg=fetusejection.

25 Dahl GJ. *Pregnancy and Childbirth Secrets*. Canada: Innovative Publishing, 2007.

26 Kirkahm M. The role of the midwife with the woman in labour: to be with, to monitor or to wait on the landing. *MIDIRS Midwifery Digest* December 2011;21(4):469-470.
27 MacLay K. The Last Taboo, *Junior Pregnancy and Baby*.
28 Buckley S. *Gentle Birth, Gentle Mothering,* Celestial Arts, 2009.
29 Buckley S, op *cit.*
30 Hayes T. 'Self-control' and the labouring woman. *MIDIRS Midwifery Digest*, September 2010;20(3):335-341.
31 Ritsuko Toda (ed). *Childbirth in Japan.* Tokyo: Birth International, 1990.
32 Wilford JN. Ancient 'birth bricks' found in Egypt. *The New York Times,* 6 August 2002. Available from: www.nytimes.com/2002/08/06/science/ancient-birth-bricks-found-in-egypt.html
33 Kitzinger S. *Rediscovering Birth.* London: Pinter and Martin, 2011.
34 Young I. *The Private Life of Islam.* London: Allen Lane, 1974; 19-20.
35 Balaskas J. *New Active Birth: A Concise Guide to Natural Childbirth.* Thorsons, 1990. First published as *Active Birth*, Unwin Paperbacks, 1983.

Chapter 5: Active management
36 O'Driscoll K, Meagher D. Active management of labor. *Clinical and Obstetric Gynecology* (supplement), Saunders, 1980.
37 McCourt C (ed). *Childbirth, Midwifery and Concepts of Time.* New York: Berghahn Books, 2010.
38 Annandale E. How midwives accomplish natural birth: managing risk and balancing expectations. *Social Problems,* 1988;35:95-110.
39 Myles MF. *A Textbook for Midwives.* 8th edn. Edinburgh: Churchill Livingstone, 1975.
40 O'Driscoll K, Meagher D, Boylan P. *Active Management of Labour.* 3rd edn. London: Mosby, 1993.
41 McCourt C. How Long Have I Got? Time in Labour: Themes from Women's Birth Stories. In: McCourt C (ed). *Childbirth, Midwifery and Concepts of Time,* New York: Berghahn Books, 2010.
42 McCourt C (ed), *op cit.*
43 Bourne G. *Pregnancy.* Pan Books, 1984.
44 Hoult IJ, MacLennan AH, Carrie LE. Lumbar epidural analgesia in labour: relation to fetal malposition and instrumental delivery. *British Medical Journal* 1977 Jan 1;1(6052):14-16.
45 Sales blurb of a drug company.
46 Enkin M, Kierse M, Neilson J, Crowther C, *et al. A Guide to Effective Care in Pregnancy and Childbirth.* Oxford: Oxford University Press, 2000.
47 Wickham S, Robinson D. Nil nocere: doing no harm as an important guiding principle within maternity care. *MIDIRS Midwifery Digest,* December 2010;20(4):415-420.
48 Kitzinger S. *Rediscovering Birth.* London: Pinter and Martin, 2011.
49 Caldeyro-Barcia R, Giussi G, Storch E, *et al.* The bearing-down efforts and their effects on fetal heart rate, oxygenation and acid base balance. *Journal of Perinatal Medicine* 1981;9 Suppl 1:63-7.
50 Masters W, Johnson V. *Masters and Johnson on Sex and Human Loving.* Little, Brown and Company, 1988.

Chapter 6: Episiotomy
51 O'Driscoll K, Meagher D, Robson M. *Active Management of Labour: The Dublin Experience.* 4th edn. Mosby, 2003.

52   Kitzinger S, ed. *Episiotomy: Physical and Emotional Aspects.* London: National Childbirth Trust, 1972.

53   Sleep J, Grant A, Garcia J *et al.* West Berkshire perineal management trial. *British Medical Journal* 1984;289(6445):587-590.

54   House M, Cario G, Jones M. Episiotomy and the perineum: a random controlled trial. *Journal of Obstetrics and Gynaecology* 2000: 96(4); 622-624.

55   Bayes S. Use of the lithotomy position for low-risk women in Perth, Australia. *British Journal of Midwifery* 2011;19(5):285-288.

56   Hofmeyr GJ, Neilson JP, Alfirevic Z, *et al. Pregnancy and Childbirth.* Chichester: Wiley and The Cochrane Collaboration, 2008.

57   Graham ID. *Episiotomy: Challenging Obstetric Intervention.* London: Blackwell Science, 1997.

58   National Collaborating Centre for Women's and Children's Health. *Intrapartum care: care of healthy women and their babies during childbirth.* Clinical Guideline commissioned by the National Institute for Health and Clinical Excellence. September 2007. Available from: http://www.nice.org.uk/nicemedia/live/11837/36275/36275.pdf.

59   Carroli G, Mignini L. Episiotomy for vaginal birth. *Cochrane Database of Systematic Reviews* 2009 Jan 21;(1):CD000081.

60   Paris AE, Greenberg JA, Ecker JL, *et al.* Is an episiotomy necessary with a shoulder dystocia? *American Journal of Obstetrics and Gynecology* 2011;205(3):217.

Chapter 7: Birth and language

61   Lerner G. *The Creation of Patriarchy.* New York: Oxford University Press, 1986:145.

62   Kitzinger S. *Rediscovering Birth.* London: Pinter & Martin, 2011.

63   Pfeufer Kahn R. *Bearing Meaning: The Language of Birth.* Chicago: University of Illinois Press, 1995.

64   Pfeufer Kahn R, *op cit;* 204.

65   Pfeufer Kahn R, *op cit;* 132.

66   *Genesis* 11:21.

67   Quoted in Pfeufer Kahn R, *op cit;* 240.

68   DeLee JB. The Prophylactic Forceps Operation, paper read before the 45th Annual Meeting of the American Gynecological Society, 24-26 May 1920, *American Journal of Obstetrics and Gynecology* 1;24-44,77-80.

69   DeLee JB, *op cit;* 1;24-44.

70   Velvovsky I, Platanov K, Ploticher V, Shugom E. *Painless Childbirth Through Psychoprophylaxis.* Moscow: Foreign Languages Publishing House, 1960.

71   Velvovsky I, *et al, op cit.*

72   Rose S. *Lifelines: Biology, Freedom, Determinism.* London: Penguin, 1998; 1-7.

73   Harris M. *An investigation of labour ward care to inform the design of a computerised decision support system for the management of childbirth.* Doctoral thesis, University of Plymouth, 2002.

74   Sherr L. *The Psychology of Pregnancy and Childbirth.* Oxford: Blackwell Science, 1995.

75   Karmel M. *Thank you, Dr Lamaze.* New York: Dolphin Books, 1965.

76   Lamaze F. *Painless Childbirth: Psychoprophylactic Method.* London: Burke, 1956.

77   Midwifery Under Threat. AIMS Journal, 21:C3; 2009. Edwards N, Murphy-Lawless J, Kirkham M, Davies S. Attacks on Midwives, Attacks on Women's Choices. *AIMS Journal* 2011 23(3). Available from: www.aims.org.uk/?Journal/Vol23No3/attacks.htm.

78   Oxorn H, Foote WR. *Human Labour and Birth.* London: Butterworths, 1968.

79   Kitzinger S. *Education and Counselling for Childbirth*. London: Bailliere Tindall, 1977.

80   Ibid.

81   Eisenberg A, Murkoff HE, Hathaway SE. *What to Expect When You're Expecting*. New York: Workman Publishing, 1991.

82   Kitzinger S. *The Experience of Childbirth*. London: Gollancz, 1962. Kitzinger S. *The New Experience of Childbirth*. London: Orion, 2004.

83   Birth Crisis Network: a phone-in helpline 01865 300266.

84   Ibid.

85   Enkin M, Keirse MJNC, Neilson J, *et al. A Guide to Effective Care in Pregnancy and Childbirth*. 3rd edn. Oxford: Oxford University Press, 2000.

86   Kitzinger S. Birth as rape: there must be an end to 'just in case' obstetrics. *British Journal of Midwifery*, Sept 2006;14(9):544-545.

87   Royal College of Obstetricians and Gynaecologists. *A career in obstetrics and gynaecology: recruitment and retention in the speciality 2006*. Available from: www.rcog.org.uk/womens-health/clinical-guidance/career-obstetrics-and-gynaecology-recruitment-and-retention-specialt.

88   Royal College of Obstetricians and Gynaecologists. *The future role of the consultant 2005*. Available from: www.rcog.org.uk/womens-health/clinical-guidance/future-role-consultant.

89   Hapangama D, Whitworth M. A career in obstetrics and gynaecology. *BMJ Career focus* 2006;333:167-169. Available from: http://careers.bmj.com/careers/advice/view-article.html?id=2007.

90   Wilkinson S, Kitzinger C. Conversation analysis, gender and sexuality. In: Weatherall A, Watson B, Gallois C, eds. *Language, Discourse and Social Psychology*. Houndmills: Palgrave Macmillan, 2007.

91   Wilkinson S, Kitzinger C. Conversation analysis. In Willig C, Stainton-Rogers W, eds. *The Handbook of Qualitative Methods in Psychology*. London: Sage, 2007.

92   Kitzinger S, Kitzinger C. *Talking with Children About Things that Matter*. London: Pandora, 1989.

Chapter 8: Birth dance

93   Raafat N. The Dance of Life. *Junior Pregnancy and Baby*, page 34. Available from: www.batterseayoga.com/pregnancy_nadia_features.htm.

94   Further information on belly dancing can be found at www.bellydancer.org.uk and www.bellydance.org.uk.

95   Al Musa M. *Dance of the Womb: The Essential Guide to Belly Dance for Pregnancy and Birth*. Byron Bay, NSW, Australia: Maha Al Musa, 2008.

96   Gaskin I. *Spiritual Midwifery*. Tennessee: The Farm, 1978.

97   Balaskas J. *Easy Exercises for Pregnancy*. London: Frances Lincoln, 1997.

Chapter 9: Water birth and song

98   Gilbert R, Tookey P. Perinatal mortality and morbidity among babies delivered in water: surveillance study and postal survey. *British Medical Journal* 1999;319;483-487.

99   Johnson P. Birth Under Water – to breathe or not to breathe, leaflet, 1995.

100   Russell K. Struggling to get into the pool room? A critical discourse analysis of labor ward midwives' experiences of water birth practices. *International Journal of Childbirth* 2011;1(1): 52-60.

101   Green JM, Coupland VA, Kitzinger JV. Expectations, experiences and psychological outcomes of childbirth: a prospective study of 825 women. *Birth* 1990;17(1):15-24.

102 Geissbühler V, Eberhard J. Waterbirths: a comparative study. A prospective study on more than 2,000 waterbirths. *Fetal Diagnosis and Therapy* 2000;15(5): 291-300.

103 Burns E, Boulton MG, Cluett E, *et al.* Characteristics, interventions, and outcomes of women who used a birthing pool: a prospective study. *Birth* September 2012;39(3):1-11.

104 Bartels Lambert. Birth songs of the Macha Galla. *Ethnology* 1969;8:406-422.

105 Beckett R. The use of music during labour and for the birth. *MIDIRS Midwifery Digest* December 2011;21(4):471-474.

Chapter 10: Home birth, midwives and doulas

106 Pilkington E. New York midwives lose right to deliver babies at home. *The Guardian*, 14 May 2010. Available from: www.guardian.co.uk/lifeandstyle/2010/may/14/home-births-new-york-midwives.

107 Royal College of Obstetricians and Gynaecologists and Royal College of Midwives. *Home Births* (Joint statement No.2). London, UK: Royal College of Midwives, April 2007. Available from: www.rcm.org.uk.

108 National Institute for Health and Clinical Excellence, National Collaborating Centre for Women's and Children's Health. *NICE clinical guideline 55: Intrapartum care*. London, UK: National Institute for Health and Clinical Excellence, September 2007:7-8. Available from: http://publications.nice.org.uk/intrapartum-care-cg55.

109 Maternity Care Working Party *Making normal birth a reality. Consensus statement from the Maternity Care Working Party: our shared views about the need to recognise, facilitate and audit normal birth.* National Childbirth Trust; Royal College of Midwives; Royal College of Obstetricians and Gynaecologists; 2007. Available from: www.rcog.org.uk/files/rcog-corp/uploaded-files/JointStatmentNormalBirth2007.pdf.

110 Declercq E, Barger M, Cabral HJ, *et al.* Maternal outcomes associated with planned primary cesarean births compared with planned vaginal births. *Obstet Gynecol* 2007;109(3):669-677.

111 Deneux-Tharaux C, Carmona E, Bouvier-Colle MH, Breart G. Postpartum maternal mortality and cesarean delivery. *Obstetrics and Gynecology* 2006;108(3 Pt 1):541-548.

112 Armstrong CA, Harding S, Matthews T, Dickinson JE. Is placenta accreta catching up with us? *Australian and New Zealand Journal of Obstetrics and Gynaecology* 2004;44(3):210-213.

113 Yang Q, Wen SW, Oppenheimer L, *et al.* Association of Caesarean delivery for first birth with placenta praevia and placental abruption in second pregnancy. *British Journal of Obstetrics and Gynaecology* 2007;114(5):609-613.

114 Smith G, Pell JP, Dobbie R. Caesarean section and risk of unexplained stillbirth in subsequent pregnancy. *Lancet* 2003;362(9398):1779-1784.

115 Gray R, Quigley MA, Hockley C, *et al.* Caesarean delivery and risk of stillbirth in subsequent pregnancy: a retrospective cohort study in an English population. *British Journal of Obstetrics and Gynaecology* 2007;114(3):264-270.

116 Shorten A, Shorten B. What happens when a private hospital comes to town? The impact of the 'public' to 'private' hospital shift on regional birthing outcomes. *Women Birth* 2007;20(2):49-55.

117 Davis J. Personal communication, 19 November, 2007.

118 Newton N. Experimental inhibition of labor through environmental disturbance. *Obstetrics and Gynecology* 1966;67:371-377.

119 Kitzinger S. Giving emotional pain a name. *The Practising Midwife* 2007;10(1):22-

23.

120 Parker, H. Personal communication, 26 November, 2007.

121 Reed B. The Albany Midwifery Practice (2). *MIDIRS Midwifery Digest* 2002;12(2):261-264.

122 Reed B. Personal communication, 26 November, 2007.

123 Page LA, McCandlish R. *The New Midwifery: Science and Sensitivity in Practice.* London: Churchill Livingstone, 2006.

124 Audit Commission. *First Class Delivery: Improving Maternity Services in England and Wales.* London: HMSO, 1997.

125 Green J, Coupland V, Kitzinger J. *Great Expectations: A Prospective Study of Women's Expectations and Experiences of Childbirth.* Cambridge: Childcare and Development Group, 1988.

126 Page L (ed). *The New Midwifery: Science and Sensitivity in Practice.* London: Churchill Livingstone, 2000.

127 Kitzinger S. Having a baby in a major teaching hospital: some women's experiences. Unpublished, 1998.

128 Kitzinger S. Foreword. In: Page L (ed). *The New Midwifery: Science and Sensitivity in Practice.* London: Churchill Livingstone, 2000.

129 Kitzinger S. *The Politics of Birth.* Oxford: Elsevier, 2005: 155-164.

130 DONA International. Standards of Practice for Birth Doulas. Available from: www.dona.org/aboutus/standards_birth.php.

131 Birth Companions: www.birthcompanions.org.uk.

132 Kitzinger S. *The Politics of Birth.* London: Elsevier, 2005.

133 Stockton A. Mindfulness and Boundaries. *Doulaing* 2008;13:19. http://doula.org.uk. Doula UK Ltd, 1 Rockfield Business Park, Old Station Drive, Leckhampton, Cheltenham, Glos GL5 0AN.

134 Film *Doulas – the Ultimate Birth Companion*, Alto Films. Available from: http://doulafilm.com.

135 Doula UK. Code of Conduct. Available from: http://doula.org.uk/content/doula-uk-code-conduct

136 Klaus M, Kennell J, Klaus P. *Mothering the Mother: How a Doula Can Help You Have a Shorter, Easier and Healthier Birth.* Cambridge, Massachusetts: Perseus Books, 1993.

137 Kitzinger S. *Rediscovering Birth.* Pinter and Martin, London, 2011.

138 Vallette C. AFP Correspondent. Press release, 24 January, 2007.

139 Doulas de France open letter of response to the press and Miviludes Commission. Available from: www.doulas.info.

140 Kirkham M. Open letter of support for doulas. Undated.

141 Osbourne J. The Roles of the Midwife and the Doula, where do they meet? *Doulaing* 13, summer 2005.

Chapter 11: Sex after the baby comes

142 Winnicott DW. *The Maturational Processes and the Facilitating Environment.* London: Hogarth, 1965.

143 Henderson BA, McMillan B, Green JM, *et al.* Men and infant feeding: perceptions of embarrassment, sexuality, and social conduct in white low-income British men. *Birth* March 2011;38(1):61-70.

144 Masters WH, Johnson VE. *Human Sexual Response.* Boston: Little Brown & Co, 1966.

145 Baxter S. Libido changes in women following first pregnancy. Unpublished. M. Phil. Dis., University of London, 1973.

146 Kenny JA. Sexuality of pregnant and breastfeeding women. *Archives of Sexual*

Behaviour 2:215-229.

147 Whitlow, D. Report of pilot survey, personal communication, Edinburgh.

148 Falicov CJ. Sexual adjustment during first pregnancy and post partum. *American Journal of Obstetrics and Gynecology* 1973;117(7):991-1000.

Chapter 12: Changing childbirth

149 Block J. *Pushed*. USA: Da Capo Press, 2007.

150 Thompson H. Promoting normal birth: appropriate use of intrapartum cardiotocography. *British Journal of Midwifery* 2011: 19(10):625-629.

151 Katz Rothman B. Address to the Midwives' Alliance of North America Conference, New York City, 1992.

152 Robinson M, Pennel CE, McLean NJ, *et al.* The over-estimation of risk in pregnancy. *Journal of Psychosomatic Obstetrics and Gynecology* 2011:32(2):53-58.

153 Evans I, Thornton H, Chalmers I. *Testing Treatments: Better Research for Better Health Care*. London: Pinter and Martin, 2010.

154 Kitzinger S. *Birth Crisis*. London: Routledge, 2006.

155 Walsh D, Downe S (eds). *Essential Midwifery Practice: Intrapartum Care*. Oxford: Blackwell, 2010.

156 Edwards N. Safety in Birth: Risk in Perspective? *Esssentially MIDIRS*, May 2011;2(5).

157 Hall MH, Ching PK, MacGillavray I. Is routine antenatal care worthwhile? *Lancet* 1980 Jul 12;2(8185):78-80.

158 Kitzinger S. *Change in antenatal care*. A report of a working party set up for the National Childbirth Trust. National Childbirth Trust, 1981.

159 Savage W. *Birth and Power: A Savage Enquiry Revisited*. London: Pinter and Martin, 2011.

160 Kitzinger S. *The Politics of Birth*. Oxford: Elsevier, 2005: 142-143.

161 Simkin P, Reinke C. *Planning Your Baby's Birth*. Seattle: Pennypress, 1980.

162 Kitzinger S. *Freedom and Choice in Childbirth*. London: Penguin, 1987.

163 Mutch L, Fawdry R. Antenatal history taking: what are we asking? *Journal of Obstetrics and Gynaecology* 1985;5(4):201-205.

164 Davidoff M, Dias T, Damus K, *et al.* Changes in the gestational age distribution among US singleton births: impact on rates of late preterm birth, 1992 to 2002. *Seminars in Perinatology* 2006;30(1): 8-15.

165 Kitzinger S. *Birth Crisis*. Abingdon: Routledge, 2006.

166 Stockton A. *Positive Pain: A Guide to Emotional Well-being through Pregnancy and Birth*. Dumfries: Solway Offset Printers, 2011.

167 Hannah ME, Hannah WJ, Hewson SA, *et al.* Planned caesarean section versus planned vaginal birth for breech presentation at term: a randomised multicentre trial. *Lancet* 356(9239):1375-83.

168 Hannah WJ. The Canadian consensus on breech management at term. *Journal of the Society of Obstetricians and Gynaecologists of Canada* 16(6):1839-48.

169 Fahy K. Is breech birth really safe?: Treatment validity in the Term Breech Trial. *Essentially MIDIRS* November 2011:2:10;17-21.

170 Banks M. *Breech birth beyond the 'Term Breech Trial'*. Birthspirit. Available from: www.birthspirit.co.nz/Articles/Articles/Breech%20birth%20beyond%20 the%20TBT.pdf.

171 Bungard T. Into the breech! *Doulaing* Autumn 2010.

INDEX